YOGA
FITNESS
FOR MEN

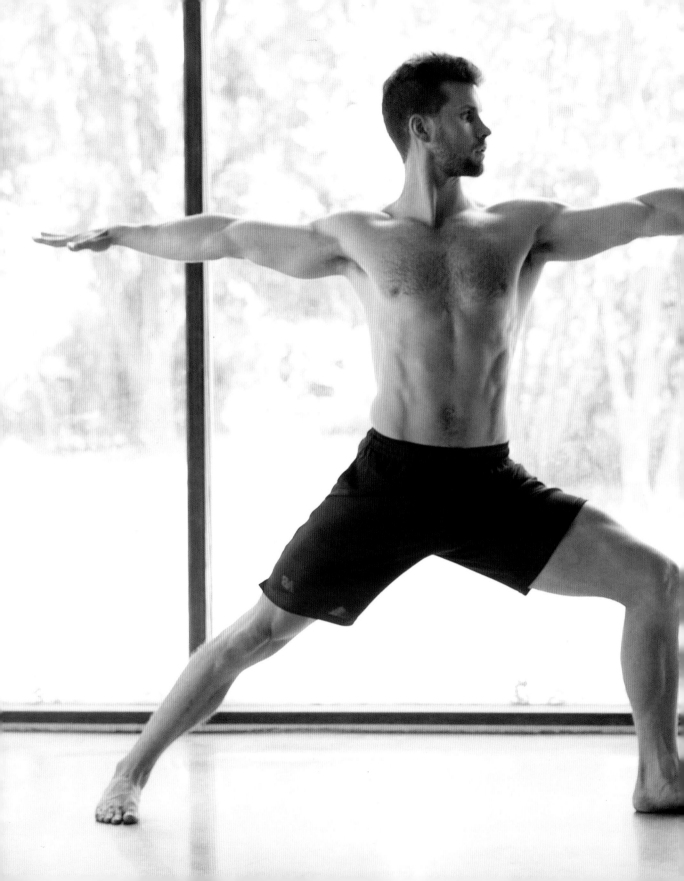

YOGA FITNESS FOR MEN

**BUILD STRENGTH
IMPROVE PERFORMANCE
INCREASE FLEXIBILITY**

DEAN POHLMAN

CONTENTS

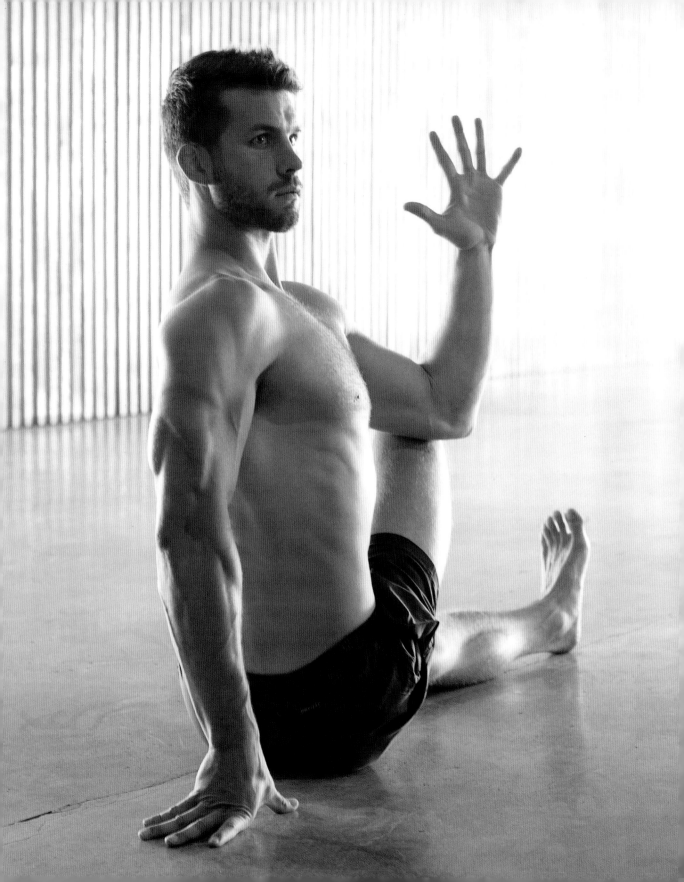

INTRODUCTION

Let's get straight to it. How can you improve your fitness with yoga? Yoga helps guys like you to move, feel, and look better. I believe in a fitness-centric approach to yoga so you can learn the techniques, understand the benefits, and know what you should (and shouldn't) be feeling in your body. That's exactly what you get in this book.

Yoga Fitness for Men was created with three types of men in mind, and there's a very good chance you identify with one of these profiles.

• **You are an athlete or fitness enthusiast** and know yoga can boost your performance. Yoga will complement your existing workout routine to make you stronger, improve your athletic performance, and prevent injury.

• **You have back, shoulder, or other joint and soft tissue problems,** and you think yoga may be able to fix your body and help you avoid more serious problems. Yoga will strengthen the areas that cause daily aches, restore a functional level of fitness, and promote both physical and mental longevity.

• **You want a sustainable fitness regimen without the stress of high-impact exercise or weights,** and you think yoga can make you stronger while being kind to your joints. Yoga will keep you active, build muscle, manage your weight, and help you feel great without the stress of cement sidewalks, plyometrics, or fast-paced weight lifting.

This book gives you the knowledge and tools to immediately begin an at-home yoga regimen, safely and effectively. It includes:

• **55 yoga postures**—step-by-step explanations of each, what you should and shouldn't be feeling, specific benefits for every posture, and modifications to meet every fitness level

• **25 workouts**—a variety of yoga routines created for your specific fitness goals, with beginner and advanced tracks

• **3 yoga programs**—structured, progressive plans that make it easy for you to start a yoga practice, and feel noticeable results in weeks, or often in just days

It doesn't matter if you're a competitive athlete or a couch potato. I wrote this book so any guy would be able to get stronger with yoga—and that includes you! If you're ready to get started, keep reading.

Dean Pohlman
Founder & CEO of Man Flow Yoga

THE BEST WORKOUT YOU'RE NOT DOING

Yoga makes you stronger in new ways by targeting aspects of fitness that traditional exercise—such as weight lifting and cardio—does not. The benefits carry over to non-physical performance areas as well, including better focus, lowered stress, and even improved internal body function. There's arguably no type of exercise that is as accessible as yoga and also effectively addresses so many aspects of your health.

BOOST ATHLETICISM

Yoga improves core strength, balance, and flexibility, all of which boost athletic performance. Whether you want better rotation for golf swings, more flexible hamstrings for smoother running, or a stronger core for more power, regularly doing yoga helps fill the gaps of your existing fitness regimen to make you a better athlete.

In addition to the physical benefits typically associated with yoga, such as flexibility, breathing, and balance, the postures also build endurance, power, and isometric strength. It's a workout that's kind to your body, particularly your joints, thanks to its no-impact nature. It's no wonder the best collegiate and professional athletes are using yoga to gain a competitive edge.

IMPROVE OVERALL HEALTH

The practice of yoga also bears non-movement benefits. If you incorporate yoga workouts regularly into your life, with patience and discipline, you'll notice a long list of benefits to your health: lowered stress, improved mental clarity, better decision-making skills, heightened quality of sleep, increased mindfulness, better body awareness, improved hormone levels (including lowered cortisol and higher testosterone), improved mood and confidence, reduced blood pressure, better immune function, and improved blood flow. The list goes on and on.

REINFORCE FUNCTIONAL MOVEMENT

Practicing yoga enables you to approach daily movement with confidence. The slow, controlled exercises improve overall muscle activation, which increases your body's mechanical efficiency. The more regular your yoga practice becomes, the stronger you get. You won't have to think about everyday movements, whether it's squatting low to pick up something off the ground, reaching for that top shelf, or bending over to tie your shoe—it will all feel natural and easy.

STRENGTHEN JOINTS AND RELIEVE ACHES

Yoga makes your muscles more mobile and flexible, relieving the pressure on your joints that causes aches and pains. It lengthens the muscles, reducing tension on the joints caused by pulling of the attached ligaments and tendons. This helps to immediately relieve discomfort, and also reduces the risk of common soft-tissue injuries in tendons, ligaments, and muscles.

Yoga even minimizes the chance of more significant injury to your spine, hips, knees, ankles, shoulders, and neck. Less pain and greater mobility are crucial for health as you age, especially if you live a mostly sedentary lifestyle. With daily practice, you'll find increased mobility through yoga is the foundation that helps you to move, feel, and even look better.

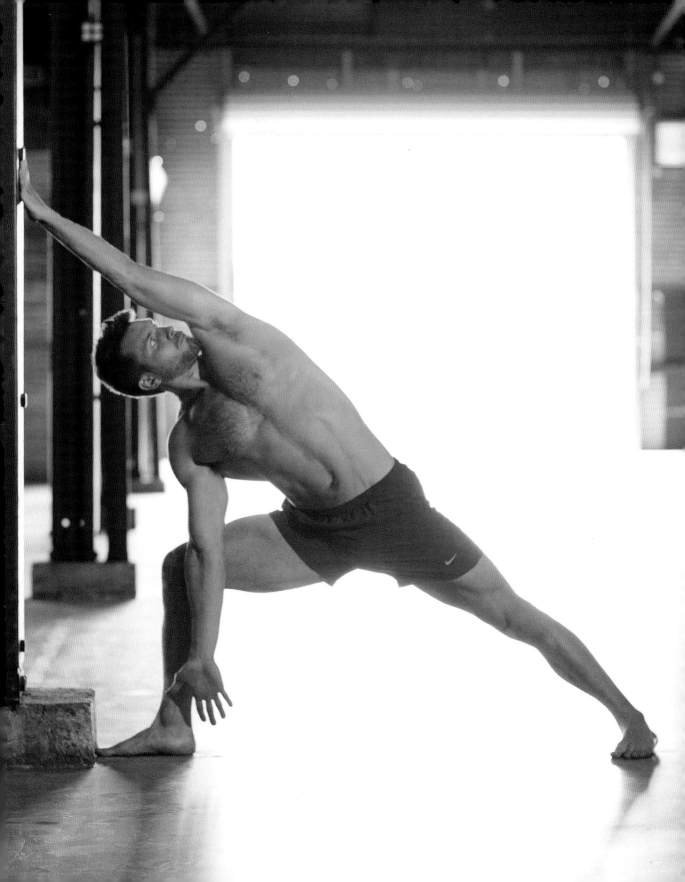

YOGA MYTHS: BUSTED

It's time to separate fact from fiction. Most of what people know about yoga is based on what they learn from popular culture, which doesn't always present an accurate picture. These pages dispel some common misconceptions that might hold you back from getting the most out of your yoga workouts.

MYTH: YOGA IS JUST STRETCHING

Some of what you do in yoga is stretching, but the majority of it is more than that. Stretching typically refers to passive lengthening of the muscles, but yoga is actually mostly active engagement. It involves balance postures, lunge and squat variations, core and spine strengthening postures, breathing work, isometric exercises, and more. Yoga combines many aspects of fitness into an efficient workout, including strength, endurance, core stability, mobility, flexibility, breathing, recovery, and, yes, stretching.

MYTH: YOGA HAS TO BE SPIRITUAL OR RELIGIOUS

The term yoga refers collectively to a group of spiritual, mental, and physical practices, but you can easily focus on just the physical aspects: the postures and the breathing. So, while yoga can be much more, it's perfectly fine to focus on the physical aspects of yoga without engaging in chanting, meditation, and spiritual practice.

MYTH: YOGA IS ONLY FOR WOMEN

It's true that three out of four people who practice yoga in the United States today are women, but the original practitioners of yoga were almost exclusively male. Yoga was practiced by men in India for thousands of years before it made its way West in the early 1900s, when it was predominantly adopted by women. However, in the early 2000s, yoga started to become popular among athletes to improve performance and prevent injury. In 2003, star NFL running back Eddie George appeared on the cover of a book called *Real Men Do Yoga*. In 2015, US professional basketball player LeBron James was leading yoga sessions at his basketball camps. In 2016, a study by Yoga Alliance found that men make up 28 percent of yoga practitioners in the United States, an increase from 20 percent in 2012. This number continues to grow, and it's now common to attend a yoga class that has as many men present as women.

MYTH: YOU CAN'T BUILD MUSCLE WITH YOGA

Wrong. Yoga actually helps you build more muscle—more efficiently, and in less time than if you were to only do resistance training. Yoga helps you directly build muscle (particularly in your back, core, hips, and thighs), but yoga really shines as an indirect method of muscle growth. It helps you regenerate muscle cells more quickly by releasing muscle tension, an essential step in the muscle-growing process. This decreases muscle recovery time and helps you get back to your workouts sooner.

Yoga also helps you avoid missing workouts due to injury, and keeps your body feeling fresh so you can stick to your workout schedule. Anyone who wants faster, more substantial muscle growth from their current workout program will benefit from regular yoga.

MYTH: I CANNOT DO YOGA BECAUSE I AM NOT FLEXIBLE

Lack of flexibility is exactly why you should do yoga. Think about it—you wouldn't avoid weights because you're not strong enough; you start lifting weights exactly because you want to get stronger, and yoga is the same. Your level of flexibility isn't what's important. It's about doing the postures in a way that works for your body and fitness level, so you can get the benefits of yoga no matter how flexible (or inflexible) you may be. All postures can be adapted to your current abilities with the right instruction and the proper tools.

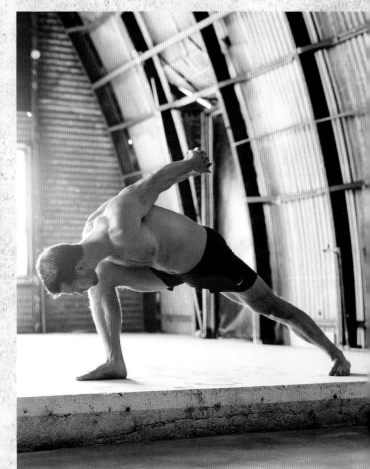

MYTH: YOU CAN'T GET INJURED DOING YOGA

Unfortunately, this is also not true. Just like any form of fitness, there is potential for injury due to incorrect technique. The most common yoga injuries result from excessive forward folds and backbends executed with poor technique, or from attempting to push your body further than it is ready to bend. But don't worry; you can reasonably expect to avoid injury by focusing on proper technique, paying attention to your body, and using common sense.

MYTH: YOGA IS THE ONLY WORKOUT I NEED TO BE HEALTHY AND STRONG

It can be, but it ultimately depends on your fitness goals and body type. Yoga is great for toning and strengthening muscles, but you may need to add resistance training like pull-ups, press-ups, or weights to your routine in order to build significant mass. Yoga also doesn't address your cardiovascular endurance, so you may want to include activities like jogging, cycling, swimming, or brisk walking in your routine to keep your heart healthy.

MYTH: YOU NEED TO PRACTICE YOGA IN THE MORNING

While morning can be a great time for yoga, it depends entirely on your schedule and preferences. You can practice any time of day. Experiment with different times to determine when is best for you. The only restriction I recommend is avoiding strenuous, strength-focused yoga workouts (or any workouts, for that matter) two to three hours before sleeping. Non-strenuous, restorative yoga, on the other hand, actually encourages better sleep and is great to do anytime in the hours leading up to bed.

THE 7 KEYS TO YOGA SUCCESS

Before you get started, learn the essential concepts for safe and effective yoga fitness. These are very important, not only because they help you do yoga more effectively and get stronger more quickly, but also because ignoring them increases your risk of injury. Internalize the seven keys as you execute your yoga practice.

1 USE SLOW, CONTROLLED MOVEMENT

Yoga can feel quite different from typical, faster-paced workouts. To get the most from your time spent on the mat, you must focus on slow, controlled movement. Follow these tips to slow down your exercise:

- **Be mindful of your body.** Notice all the little things, such as what each muscle is doing, body positioning, breathing, and tension you may or may not be holding on to.
- **Little changes make the difference.** Make subtle adjustments to improve technique. Moving just a centimeter can feel different.
- **Listen to your body.** Pay attention to the sensations of stretching and muscle engagement. Use your intuition to determine when to push a little more, or to back off.

2 CONTROL YOUR BREATH, CONTROL YOUR BODY

This is one of the most important aspects of yoga. Controlling your breath makes your yoga workout more effective by allowing you to hold the postures for a longer time, relax more easily into the postures, and work deeper into your mobility. It also helps with innumerable non-performance aspects of fitness, such as decreased anxiety, better sleep, lowered stress, and even weight loss. Remember these breathing techniques every time you practice:

- **Match your breaths with your movements.** As you inhale, lengthen your body, and as you exhale, work deeper into the posture.

- **Slow down your breathing.** If you're a beginner, start with 3-second inhales and exhales. If you're more advanced, work your way up to 5- or 6-second inhales and exhales.
- **Take longer breaths in restorative poses.** It's easier to breathe longer in these types of postures, which will help you relax and go deeper. Try to work up to 10-second breaths.

3 ENGAGE YOUR CORE

This refers to engagement of the body's core muscles, made up of the muscles in the front, back, and sides of the body's mid-section. Every posture you do in yoga should involve active core engagement. Core muscles form the power center of your body, helping you produce explosive movements, protect your spine, create stability for balance, and help with just about any full-body movement you can imagine. A weak core significantly increases the risk of injury in your spine, knees, hips, and shoulders.

Use this simple technique to understand what proper core engagement feels like: stand tall, take a deep breath in, then slowly exhale all the air from your lungs. The tightening feeling you have in the muscles surrounding your belly is core engagement. Incorporate this feeling into every posture you do. It won't be perfect at first, and you'll probably forget to do it often, but eventually core engagement will become a habit that you will not even have to think about.

4 RELAX—IT'S YOGA

One incredibly important aspect of yoga is relaxing your body. Even in the most intense postures, strive to stay relaxed by maintaining composure and keeping your breathing long. This not only helps you maintain the posture for a longer time, but it also helps you work deeper into mobility, develop body awareness, lower anxiety and stress, and more. It's what makes yoga, yoga. Consider the following to help relax:

- **Slow down your breathing.** This enables your muscles to release tension and lengthen.
- **Release tension in commonly tense areas.** Your neck, shoulders, and facial expressions all affect stress in the rest of the body.
- **Relax your mind.** In other words, don't think about everything on your to-do list, or whatever else bothers you that day. This creates unneeded stress and makes it difficult to relax. Instead, focus intently on your breath and body.

5 MAKE IT WORK FOR YOU; DO NOT JUST MIRROR OTHERS

Form is important, but you have to do each posture in a way that's appropriate for your body, rather than just copying someone else. Everyone has varying levels of strength and mobility, which means proper technique for one person might not look the same for you. Here are some guidelines to make sure you're doing the pose to match your body and fitness level:

- **Focus on achieving the correct sensations in your body,** including the appropriate stretching and muscle engagement for the posture.
- **Use the posture instructions** in this book for thorough, specific guidance on what you should and should not feel.
- **Modify as needed.** Use blocks or a strap to facilitate the proper sensations. These are tools, not crutches, so use them as often as you would like.

6 ACCEPT THAT IT'S A DIFFERENT KIND OF PUSH

In other workouts, it may help to push harder, grit your teeth, and tense your muscles, but that won't get you very far in yoga. Yoga is all about establishing control over your body. Here are the main ways to do that:

- **Relax into the discomfort.** Use mental focus to hold on for just a few more breaths to work a little bit deeper, all while maintaining control.
- **Constantly refine your technique.** Are your knees in the right position? Are your ankles and shoulders doing what they should? Go through a mental checklist from head to toe every time you do a posture, and keep cycling through that checklist until it's time for the next posture.
- **Tease your flexibility limits.** This is the yoga equivalent of pushing yourself to finish the last two reps. It's where the growth happens. If you want to get stronger with yoga, you should become accustomed to working into this zone of safe discomfort. However, be careful; you can get injured if you push too far.

7 BUILD A PRACTICE

Doing yoga every now and then won't cut it. In order to reap the benefits, you need to do yoga at least two or three times per week. It is important to practice consistently, in terms of both effort and frequency. Be sure to:

- **Set a manageable schedule for yourself.** Within a few weeks, it will become a habit, not just because it's on the calendar, but because you'll start to notice a difference and won't want to stop.
- **Do every routine the best you can on every given day.** Maybe your muscles are sore, or you didn't sleep well last night. The point is you don't always feel 100 percent, so you should only expect to do as well as you can according to how you feel at the time. This is not only sensible, but it also delivers better long-term results. Your body needs rest—even from yoga!

MINDFUL EXERCISE

One reason yoga is so different from other types of movement is the slow, or often static, nature of the exercises. In order to notice significant results and avoid injury, you need to pay close attention to your body, especially proper physical alignment and technique. Every posture involves stretching, muscle engagement, and spinal alignment—review these before you get started.

High lunge pose has elements of both muscle engagement and stretching.

Stretch in shoulders

Engagement of core

Stretch in right hip flexors

Engagement of right quadriceps, glutes, and hip flexors

Engagement of left quadriceps, glutes, and hamstrings

MUSCLE ENGAGEMENT VERSUS STRETCHING

These opposing forces are present in almost every yoga posture. You simultaneously lengthen (stretch) one group of muscles, while you flex (engage and shorten) the opposing muscle group.

Muscle engagement refers to an increase in muscular tension. It's the tightening feeling in your muscles when you lift, push, or pull. Think of muscle engagement as strength; it's what allows your body to do basic work, such as lifting objects, standing up from a seated position, or pushing a piece of furniture across the floor. Ability to engage your muscles is a combination of motor control and muscular strength. Motor control is the process by which your brain activates and coordinates your muscles, while muscular strength is the ability of the muscle to create and sustain tension.

Stretching refers to positions that decrease tension and lengthen muscles. It aids recovery, relieves stiffness, and reduces tension on joints, ligaments, and tendons. It's the feeling in your hamstrings when you reach to touch your toes, or the sensation in your sides when

SPINAL ALIGNMENTS

There are three primary types of spinal alignment in yoga (not including bending to the side or twisting). Put these concepts into practice as you perform all yoga postures.

NEUTRAL ALIGNMENT

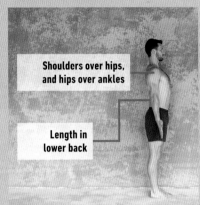

Shoulders over hips, and hips over ankles

Length in lower back

FLEXION

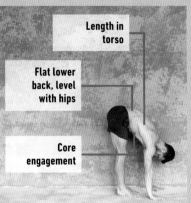

Length in torso

Flat lower back, level with hips

Core engagement

EXTENSION

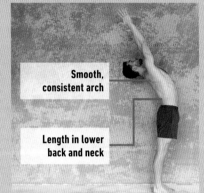

Smooth, consistent arch

Length in lower back and neck

Neutral alignment is the position of your spine in perfect standing posture. It isn't totally straight; it curves inward at your lower back and neck, and outward at the mid-back, to form an S-curve.

Be sure to: engage core, hips, and thighs; keep length in lower back by reaching tailbone toward the floor

Flexion is when the spine is rounded, called a forward fold position in yoga. When done properly, poses involving spinal flexion stretch the back of your body while strengthening the front of the body.

Be sure to: lengthen front of torso; engage abs and hip flexors; avoid rounding lower back (use a block or bend knees, if needed)

Extension is when your spine is arched, called a backbend in yoga. To protect the spine in extension, the abdominal and hip muscles, as well as the muscles surrounding the spine, should be completely engaged.

Be sure to: engage core and back of neck; avoid over-arching lower back and neck; keep hips neutral; focus on length, not depth

---

you reach overhead. Ability to stretch isn't just muscular. It also depends on your ability to relax, joint range of motion, and body temperature.

Most postures are a combination of engagement and stretching. While one muscle engages, the opposing muscle stretches. Generally speaking, the postures that involve engagement, or a combination of engagement and stretching, are considered strength-focused exercises. Postures involving only stretching are considered restorative.

MOBILITY VERSUS FLEXIBILITY

In this book, mobility is an umbrella term that includes flexibility.

Flexibility is passive range of motion; before you can use your muscles to place your body in certain positions, you need the passive capacity to get into that position. Using an external force, such as your arm or a strap, creates a passive stretch where the stretched muscles are just along for the ride.

Mobility is active muscle engagement within range of motion. Standing on one leg and lifting the other leg to hip level is mobility. Flexibility precedes mobility, but in order to improve athletic performance, you should strive for mobility.

START SMART

Yoga is most effective when you practice it consistently and with purpose. This book includes all of the information, tools, and tips you need to get started. Here's how to use this book to intelligently begin your yoga practice.

1 LEARN THE 7 KEY CONCEPTS

The first step is understanding the overarching concepts that allow you to safely and effectively practice yoga. It's important to understand what you should be focusing on while practicing so that you get stronger as efficiently as possible, while avoiding injury. Yoga is different from other workouts, and many concepts may seem unfamiliar (maybe even counterintuitive), so review the key concepts on pages 12 and 13 before performing any postures.

WORKOUTS

Choose from 3 workout categories, described on p128

2 SELECT A WORKOUT OR PROGRAM

This book has 25 stand-alone workouts and 3 longer-term programs. Workouts are sequences of yoga postures that address specific needs, such as building core strength or relieving neck pain. The long-term programs give you specific workouts to complete on a daily basis for months at a time, ensuring that your hard work will pay off. To help you select a program, read the descriptions starting on page 182.

PROGRAMS

Select 1 of 3 programs tailored to your goals

Identifies who the program can best benefit

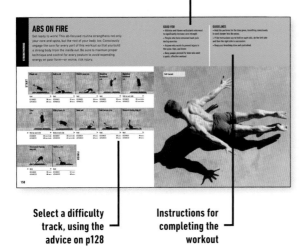

Select a difficulty track, using the advice on p128

Instructions for completing the workout

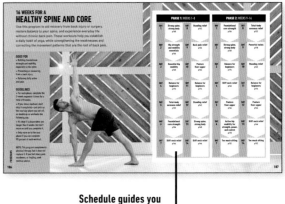

Schedule guides you through each day of the program

GET YOUR GEAR

All you need is a mat, but you will have a more effective session if you also have one or two yoga blocks and a yoga strap—these help you tailor the poses to your body. Cork blocks will provide more stability than foam ones. For the strap, use any that won't irritate your skin. A rope or belt works, too.

3 EXPLORE THE POSTURES

It's important to familiarize yourself with the postures before you start. First, read all of the instructional text, then try the pose for yourself, making sure to follow all technique prompts. Now you're ready to start the workout. After all, you learn best by doing, so you can now put the book down and get to work.

POSTURES

55 thorough guides for each yoga pose

Cues for what you should and should not be feeling

Alternative views make sure you see all helpful angles

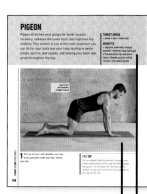
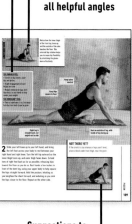

Visual, step-by-step instruction with annotations so you know exactly what to do

Suggestions to modify the pose so it's just right for you

Primary benefits of each pose are highlighted

FINAL ADVICE FROM DEAN

What's the secret to working out? This book has all the tools you need—yoga concepts, postures, and workouts—but there's a few more lessons to help you form a successful practice. Implementing these simple ideas helps you form unbreakable habits to accomplish your goals.

1 **Identify your real reason for working out,** and make that the basis of everything you do. There's a reason why you work out, one that is really driving you. Whatever it is, figure it out! Then create goals for yourself based around this reason and select workouts and programs that reflect those goals. Constantly remind yourself why you began, and you'll see substantial results.

• **Tired of chronic back pain?** Think of how great it will be to move without pain.

• **Want to be a better athlete?** Keep in mind the performance increases you can look forward to.

• **Want to look better in the mirror?** Think about the dream body you've always wanted.

2 **Set a schedule and stick to it.** Many people get to the gym and aren't sure what they're going to do. They spend half their time just thinking about the exercises they'll do, instead of spending that energy on the workouts themselves. Plan your workout ahead of time, being as specific as you can. This frees up your energy for the workout itself, rather than on trying to figure it out.

3 **Keep a record of your workouts** to hold yourself accountable and track your training. A complete log helps you to understand your fitness because you can look back and see what you were doing two months ago and compare that to what you're doing now. More than that, it's a physical representation of all the hard work and time you put into your goals. It's something to take pride in. I recommend buying a small journal for this, and not using it for anything else.

1 POSTURES

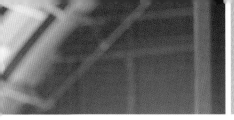

Learn the postures to practice yoga safely and effectively. This section includes a thorough guide of 55 yoga poses, explained in beginner's terms.

Each posture includes the following:

Target areas
Understand the target muscle groups and body parts for each pose, and choose the postures your body needs.

Benefits
How does this make me stronger? How does that relieve pain or prevent injury? Learn how each pose improves your fitness.

Step-by-step technique
Get stronger more quickly, and avoid injury. Learn what each part of your body should be doing for every pose.

What you should feel and shouldn't feel
Understand what you should be feeling in your body; as well as what you should not be feeling, and how to fix it.

Not there yet? and Pro tip
Pick the variation for you. Choose an easier modification if the pose is too difficult, or look at the tip if it's too easy.

MOUNTAIN

This basic standing pose is the foundation upon which all other yoga postures are built. Mastering this posture and applying it to everyday movement is one of the most beneficial practices you can do for your body. Mountain builds body awareness, improves breathing, and even boosts your confidence.

TARGET AREA
• total body

BENEFITS
• Corrects posture • Highlights muscle imbalances • Prepares you for your workout • Improves confidence • Relieves anxiety

1 Stand with your big toes touching and your heels about 1in (2.5cm) apart. Press down through your heels, balls of the feet, and big toes. Gently squeeze your inner thighs and hips toward each other. Lift your sternum and the crown of your head toward the ceiling. Hold your arms at your sides, palms facing forward. Inhale as you expand your chest (making sure not to lift the shoulders), and exhale as you empty your lungs and squeeze navel to spine.

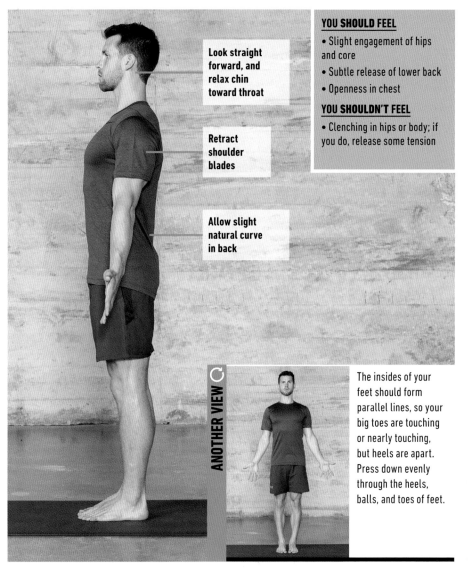

Look straight forward, and relax chin toward throat

Retract shoulder blades

Allow slight natural curve in back

YOU SHOULD FEEL
• Slight engagement of hips and core
• Subtle release of lower back
• Openness in chest

YOU SHOULDN'T FEEL
• Clenching in hips or body; if you do, release some tension

ANOTHER VIEW

The insides of your feet should form parallel lines, so your big toes are touching or nearly touching, but heels are apart. Press down evenly through the heels, balls, and toes of feet.

PRO **TIP**
Avoid leaning forward onto the balls of your feet and toes; keep weight centered. Close your eyes to work on your body awareness and balance.

STANDING FORWARD FOLD

This posture actively stretches your hamstrings to release tension in your spine and back. Focus on engaging the correct muscles to stretch the hamstrings, and don't worry about whether you can touch your hands to the floor. This posture is great after a workout or long walk.

TARGET AREAS
• hamstrings • core • mid-back
• upper back

BENEFITS
• Improves hamstring flexibility
• Relieves tension in entire spine
• Prevents soft-tissue injuries in hips and thighs

1 Stand in Mountain (see p20) with your big toes touching and heels about 1in (2.5cm) apart. Inhale to lift arms overhead, then exhale as you hinge at the hips and squeeze torso toward upper thighs. Let fingertips move toward the floor. Tuck chin to chest, looking backward to lengthen back of neck. Maintain a flat back by firmly engaging abs and squeezing inner thighs. Hold the posture, inhaling as you lengthen the spine, and exhaling as you fold deeper.

PRO **TIP**
Actively flex the muscles in the front of the body to feel the stretch in the back of the body. Focus on keeping the back flat. Bend knees as necessary; hamstring flexibility comes with time.

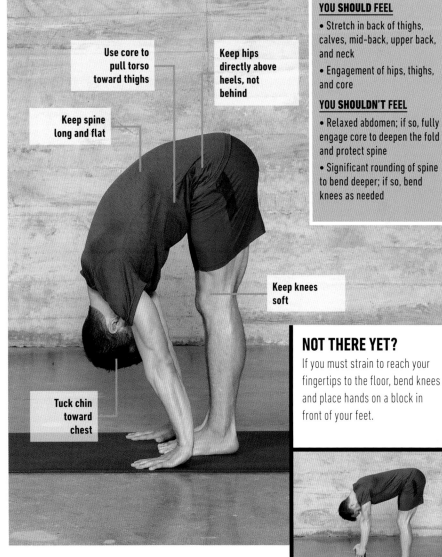

Use core to pull torso toward thighs

Keep hips directly above heels, not behind

Keep spine long and flat

Keep knees soft

Tuck chin toward chest

YOU **SHOULD FEEL**
• Stretch in back of thighs, calves, mid-back, upper back, and neck
• Engagement of hips, thighs, and core

YOU **SHOULDN'T FEEL**
• Relaxed abdomen; if so, fully engage core to deepen the fold and protect spine
• Significant rounding of spine to bend deeper; if so, bend knees as needed

NOT THERE YET?
If you must strain to reach your fingertips to the floor, bend knees and place hands on a block in front of your feet.

HALF LIFT

This is a fantastic posture for relieving back pain, and it's a great way to warm up your spine for yoga practice, making it an essential part of vinyasa or "flow" yoga classes. If you're a beginner, allow your knees to bend, and use a block to reach the ground.

TARGET AREAS
• hamstrings • core • spine

BENEFITS
• Improves hamstring mobility
• Reduces risk of spine and hip injury • Relieves back pain caused by tight hips

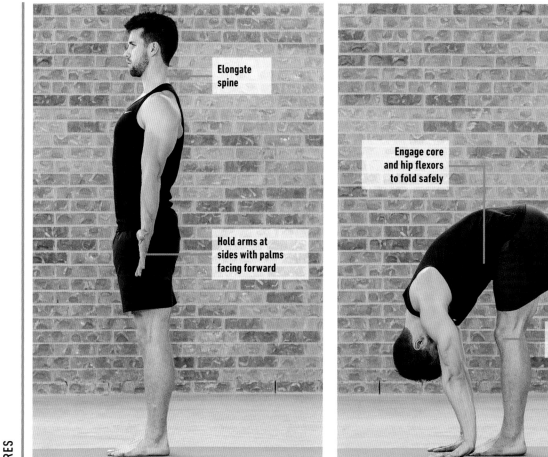

Elongate spine

Hold arms at sides with palms facing forward

Engage core and hip flexors to fold safely

Keep soft bend in knees

1 Stand in Mountain pose (see p20) with your big toes touching and your heels about 1in (2.5cm) apart.

2 Hinge at the hips, pulling your chest toward your thighs, and your thighs toward your chest, to move into Standing forward fold (see p21).

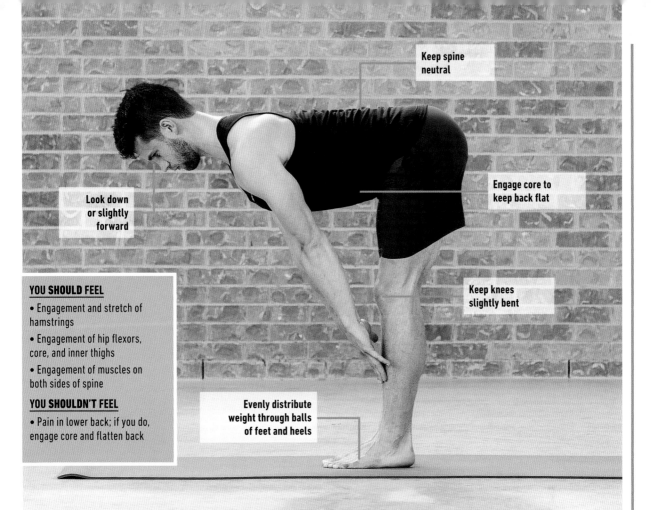

Keep spine neutral

Engage core to keep back flat

Look down or slightly forward

Keep knees slightly bent

YOU SHOULD FEEL
• Engagement and stretch of hamstrings
• Engagement of hip flexors, core, and inner thighs
• Engagement of muscles on both sides of spine

YOU SHOULDN'T FEEL
• Pain in lower back; if you do, engage core and flatten back

Evenly distribute weight through balls of feet and heels

3 Inhale as you pull your torso forward and up, making your spine straight and parallel to the floor. Lightly press hands into your shins to lengthen chest forward. Reach tailbone upward and tighten your abs to straighten your spine. Engage your thighs by lightly squeezing your legs toward each other. Hold the posture, inhaling as you lengthen the spine, and exhaling as you tighten the core and stretch the hamstrings.

PRO **TIP**
Imagine yourself tipping forward slightly—this helps you properly engage your core, strengthen your spine, and work deeper into the hamstrings.

NOT THERE YET?
If you can't keep your back straight, rest your hands on a block in front of you, and bend your knees as needed.

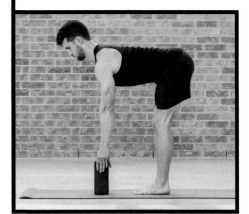

HALF SUN SALUTATION

This three-posture series is a shortened version of a traditional yoga flow, or sequence of postures linked by transitional movements. This flow is a great warm up to activate and open the muscles in the whole body. If it is difficult to combine the breathing with the movements, practice just the movements first.

TARGET AREAS
• spine • arms • legs

BENEFITS
• Activates total body • Releases spinal tension • Relaxes muscles when you're stiff or sore

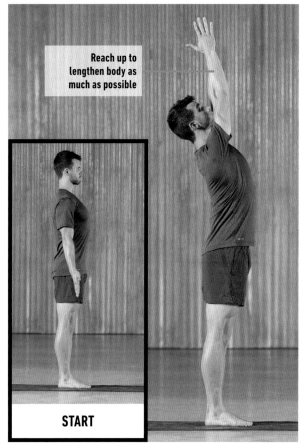

Reach up to lengthen body as much as possible

START

1 Start in Mountain pose (see p20) with big toes touching and arms at your sides, palms facing forward. Inhale as you sweep your arms out to the sides and overhead, bringing palms together and looking up at your hands.

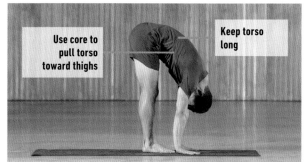

Use core to pull torso toward thighs

Keep torso long

2 Exhale as you hinge at the hips and sweep your arms wide, down to Standing forward fold (see p21), slightly bending your knees and relaxing your hands toward the floor. Keep core actively engaged. Tuck chin to look behind you.

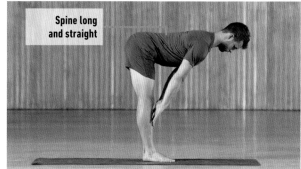

Spine long and straight

3 Inhale to pull your chest forward and lift your torso to Half lift (see p22), forming an L-shape with your body. Lightly press hands to your shins, making back parallel to floor. Tuck chin toward throat, and look straight down.

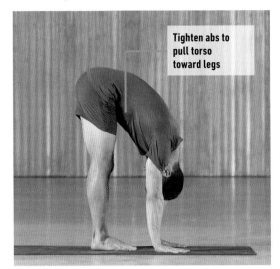

Tighten abs to pull torso toward legs

4 Exhale as you lower your torso back to Standing forward fold (see p21) by hinging at the hips and reaching your hands to the floor. Use your core to pull torso toward thighs. This fold should feel deeper than the first one.

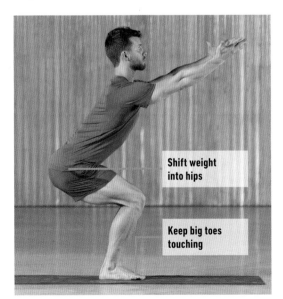

Shift weight into hips

Keep big toes touching

5 Lower your hips as if sitting down onto a chair, and use your core to lift your chest away from your thighs. Sweep arms out wide, palms facing the ceiling.

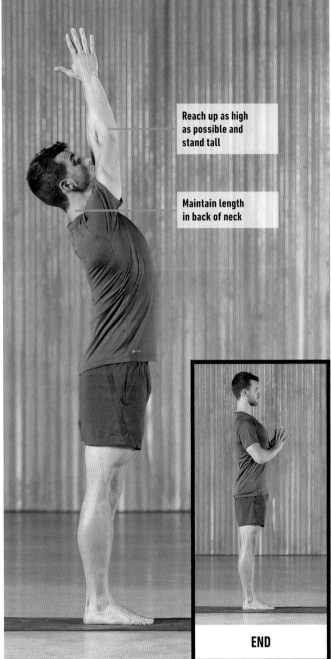

Reach up as high as possible and stand tall

Maintain length in back of neck

END

6 Inhale deeply as you press down through your heels, extending hands as high as possible to stand as tall as you can, and pressing palms firmly together overhead. To end, exhale as you bring your hands to your sternum (called the "heart center" in yoga).

WIDE-LEGGED FORWARD FOLD

This position stretches your inner thighs, relieves tension in your back, and helps prevent knee injuries. It's an essential cool-down posture for athletes because it promotes speedy recovery and improves lateral mobility. Wide-legged forward fold is also ideal for any person fighting chronic lower-back pain.

TARGET AREAS
• inner thighs • hamstrings • ankles

BENEFITS
• Prevents soft-tissue injury in thighs and hips • Speeds inner-thigh and hamstring recovery • Strengthens knees • Relieves lower-back tension

1 Stand with your feet 4 to 6ft (1.25–1.75m) apart, and slightly turn your toes inward. Engage the arches of your feet, and press into outer edges of feet.

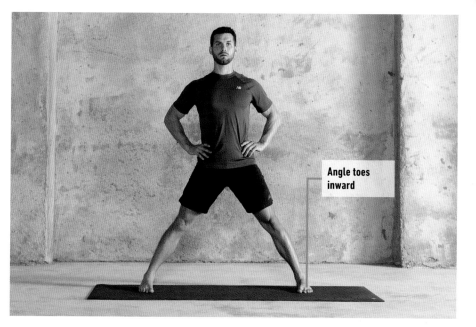

Angle toes inward

2 Engage your quadriceps and squeeze your inner thighs toward each other. Hinge at the hips and pull your chest forward and down, maintaining a flat back. Rest your fingers on the floor below your shoulders.

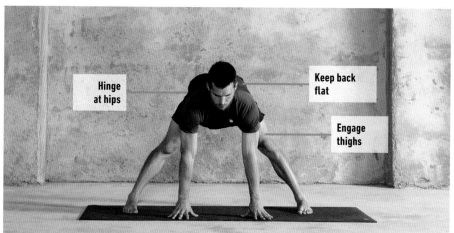

Hinge at hips

Keep back flat

Engage thighs

- Stretch in inner thighs, hamstrings, and outer ankles
- Release in back
- Engagement of hip flexors, thighs, and core

YOU **SHOULDN'T FEEL**
- Significantly rounded back; if so, pull chest forward and don't fold as deep
- Hips relaxing backward; if so, bring them slightly forward

Keep abdomen long and engaged to protect lower back

Continue to engage thighs

Keep weight in outsides of feet

3 Squeeze hip flexors and core toward each other, and fold forward as far as you can while keeping the back flat. Hold the posture, inhaling as you pull your chest forward and lengthen the body, and exhaling as you fold deeper.

PRO **TIP**

Add a chest stretch by interlacing your fingers behind your back and lifting arms away from your back, as in Humble warrior (see p42). You could also hold either end of a strap, rather than interlacing your fingers.

NOT THERE YET?

If your back is rounding, bend knees, and rest your hands on a block in front of you.

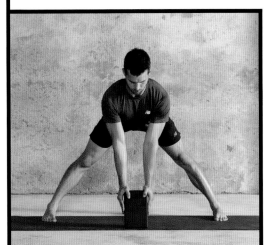

STANDING BACKBEND

This posture is extremely effective for strengthening the core and spine, and for improving spinal mobility. Use it in the morning to wake up with an energy boost. Standing backbend is also great before a workout to activate your core and warm up your spine.

TARGET AREAS
• core • spine • shoulders

BENEFITS
• Strengthens spine and core
• Corrects posture • Improves balance and spinal mobility
• Opens chest

1 Stand in Mountain pose (see p20) with your big toes touching and your heels about 1in (2.5cm) apart. Reach your arms overhead, press palms together, and interlace fingers, pointing the index fingers up.

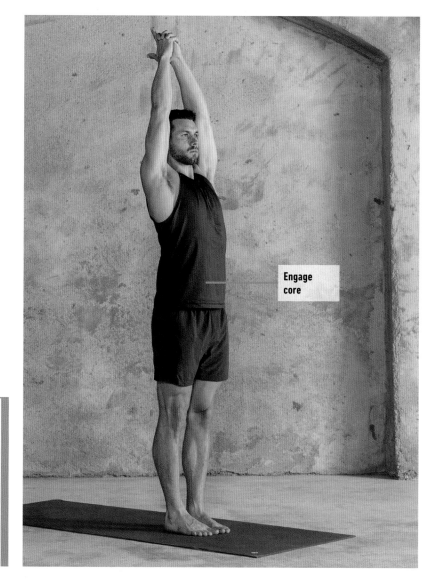

Engage core

PRO **TIP**

This pose is a constant push and pull between lengthening the spine and deepening the arch. As you inhale, lengthen the spine and grow taller. As you exhale, increase the degree of the backbend and reach further back.

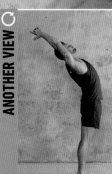
Bend back only as far as it feels comfortable and core remains engaged. Do not let your lower back arch.

YOU SHOULD FEEL
• Stretch through chest and shoulders

YOU SHOULDN'T FEEL
• Neck pain; if you do, keep the back of neck long and engaged
• Lower-back pain; if you do, reach tailbone down, and increase core engagement

Keep core engaged

Keep hips over ankles

Lock knees

NOT THERE YET?
Extend your arms without interlacing your fingers.

Press evenly through feet

2 Inhale as you slowly look up at the ceiling, then exhale as you bend backward. Keep hips and core engaged, and maintain length in your spine. Hold the posture, inhaling as you lengthen the spine and lift the sternum higher, and exhaling as you bend deeper and reach further back.

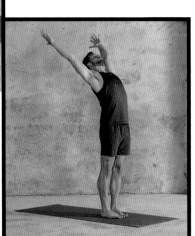

STANDING BACKBEND

STANDING SIDEBEND

This sidebend strengthens your shoulders and core while improving mobility in the shoulders and sides of your body. This posture is also important for increasing spinal mobility and relieving tension in your spine and hips. Start with a shallow bend, and focus on feeling the stretch in the correct areas.

TARGET AREAS
• shoulders • core • spine
• side body

BENEFITS
• Improves shoulder mobility and health • Corrects posture
• Increases upper-body strength and endurance

1 Stand in Mountain pose (see p20) with your big toes nearly touching and your heels about 1in (2.5cm) apart. Interlace your fingers overhead. Lock your arms, and point your index fingers to the ceiling.

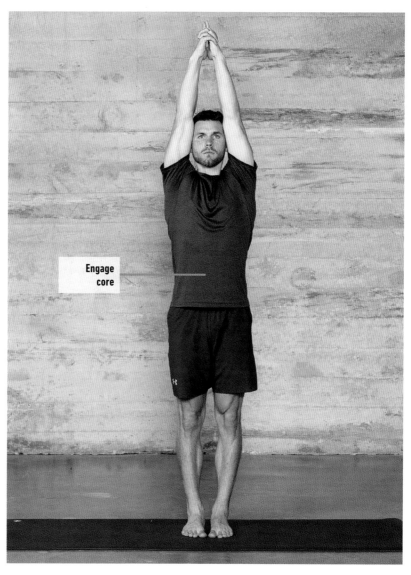

Engage core

PRO **TIP**
For better core stability, squeeze your thighs toward one another, and engage the muscles in the side of the body that you are stretching.

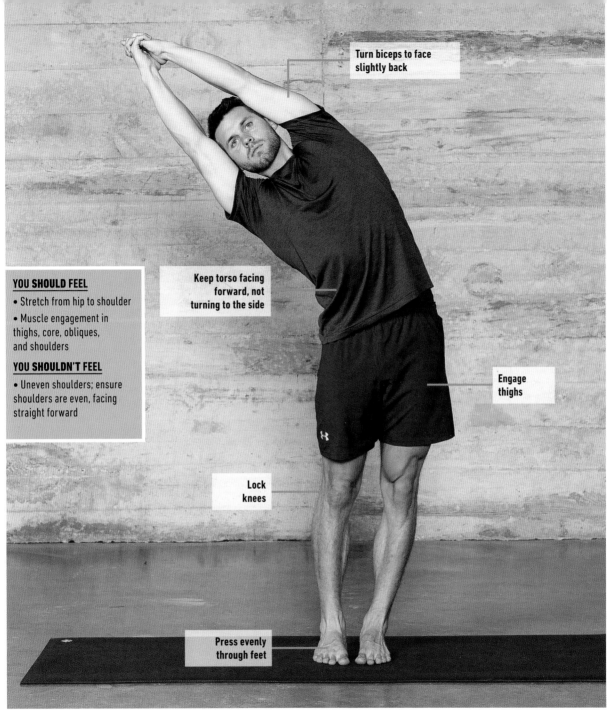

Turn biceps to face slightly back

Keep torso facing forward, not turning to the side

Engage thighs

Lock knees

Press evenly through feet

YOU SHOULD FEEL
- Stretch from hip to shoulder
- Muscle engagement in thighs, core, obliques, and shoulders

YOU SHOULDN'T FEEL
- Uneven shoulders; ensure shoulders are even, facing straight forward

2 Rotate your arms inward so your biceps face your ears. Press down into the heels and the balls of your feet. Make your body as tall as possible, then lean to the right with your upper body, hips lightly pressing in the opposite direction. Hold the posture, inhaling as you get taller, and exhaling as you bend deeper. Repeat on the left side.

CHAIR

This basic yoga squat is perfect for runners, people who sit often, and anyone who wants to have better workouts. Chair develops muscle activation in your glutes, improving your squats, lunges, and sprints. It also prevents lower-back pain and strengthens your knees.

TARGET AREAS
• glutes • hips • thighs • ankles

BENEFITS
• Improves hip strength and muscle activation • Addresses cause of exercise-induced lower-back pain • Activates lower-body muscles • Improves ankle mobility for squats

1 Stand in Mountain pose (see p20) with your big toes touching and your heels about 1in (2.5cm) apart. Reach your arms overhead, palms facing inward. Squeeze thighs toward each other, and engage your abdominal muscles.

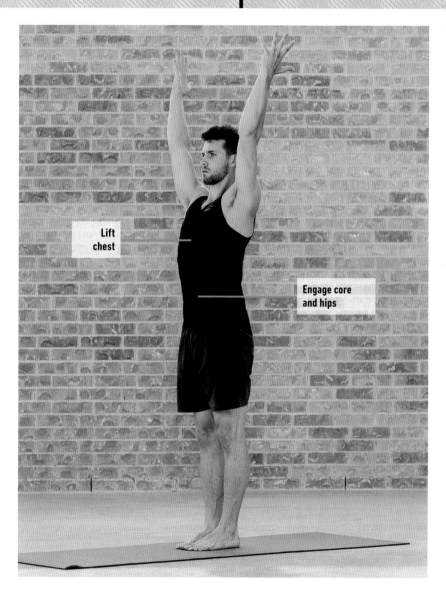

Lift chest

Engage core and hips

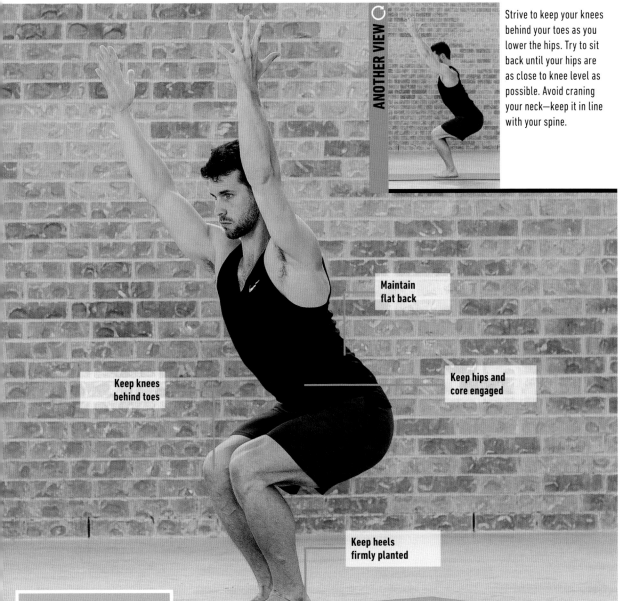

Strive to keep your knees behind your toes as you lower the hips. Try to sit back until your hips are as close to knee level as possible. Avoid craning your neck—keep it in line with your spine.

Maintain flat back

Keep knees behind toes

Keep hips and core engaged

Keep heels firmly planted

YOU SHOULD FEEL
- Stretch in shoulders
- Engagement of glutes, thighs, lower legs, and core

YOU SHOULDN'T FEEL
- Your body leaning forward; if so, raise hips higher, flatten back, and sink down again
- Strain in knees; if you do, shift weight to hips

2 Slowly bend your knees and lower your hips down and back, as if sitting down onto a chair. Keep your arms overhead and rotated inward so your biceps face back. Keep your center of gravity in your hips and core, not in knees. Maintain height in torso and avoid collapsing your chest. Keep spine neutral. Hold the posture, inhaling to maintain length, and exhaling to sit deeper.

DEEP SQUAT

No matter your fitness aspirations, every person can benefit from an improved squat technique—it's the most important of all lower-body exercises. Deep squat will build core and hip strength, improve hip and ankle mobility, and prevent pain or injury in your spine and knees. Squat daily!

TARGET AREAS
• hips • core • ankles • thighs

BENEFITS
• Improves hip power, strength, and endurance • Builds functional core strength • Strengthens spine and prevents lower-back pain

1 Stand with your feet shoulder-width apart, toes facing straight forward. (It's okay to angle toes slightly outward at first, if needed.) Slightly arch your lower back. Raise arms to shoulder height, palms facing the ceiling.

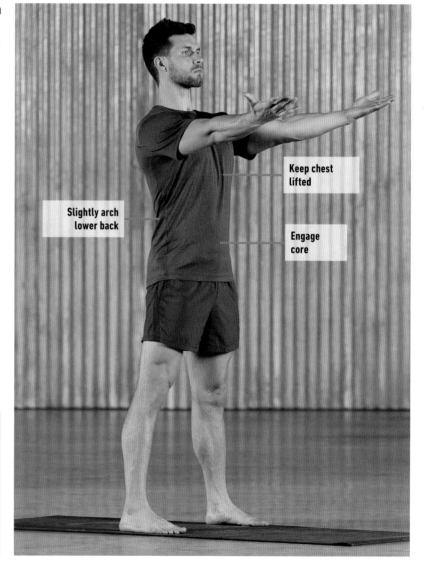

Slightly arch lower back

Keep chest lifted

Engage core

PRO **TIP**
Once you are in the squat, lightly press your hands into inner thighs to lift torso away from thighs and push knees outward. This helps strengthen the core more.

YOU **SHOULD FEEL**
• Engagement of glutes, hips, and core

YOU **SHOULDN'T FEEL**
• Weight shifted forward in knees; if you do, shift weight back into hips
• Tension in knees; if you do, push hips further back, and squeeze glutes and inner thighs

Allow slight arch in back

Lift chest away from thighs

Push knees out, slightly wider than ankles

Squeeze glutes together

NOT THERE YET?
If it is difficult to remain upright while arching your back and squatting, hold on to a sturdy external support, and use it to lean back and sit deeper.

Keep weight back in heels and hips

2 Keeping your chest upright, slowly lower your hips down and back into a squat until hips are just below the knees. Press down firmly through your heels, the balls of your feet, and your toes. Drive knees outward to engage glutes. Keep arms extended in front of you to maintain balance. Hold the posture, inhaling as you lift the chest and get taller, and exhaling as you sit deeper.

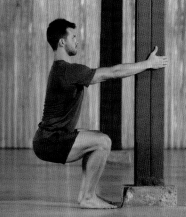

HORSE

Also called Goddess, this is a fantastic pose to build groin mobility and hip strength. This squat isolates the glutes to reduce the risk of knee injury, correct muscle imbalances in runners, and improve hip mobility in all athletes for better performance. Horse also addresses the root of back pain caused by excessive sitting.

TARGET AREAS
• hips • core • groin • glutes

BENEFITS
• Strengthens lower body • Improves hip mobility to prevent soft-tissue injury • Increases range of motion for kicking, squats, and changes of direction

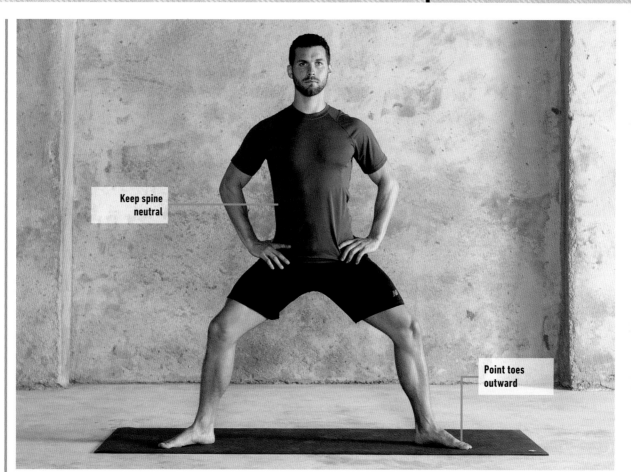

Keep spine neutral

Point toes outward

1 Stand with your feet 3 to 4ft (1–1.25m) apart. Turn your toes out to at least 45 degrees, but up to 90 degrees as able. Place hands on your hips to help maintain neutral alignment.

PRO **TIP**
Gluteal engagement makes this pose effective at increasing groin mobility. Pretend you are squeezing a coin between your glutes, and sink deeper.

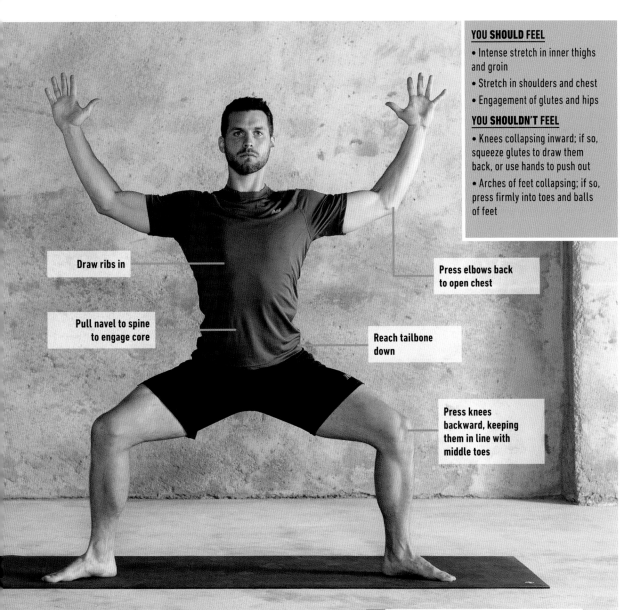

• Intense stretch in inner thighs and groin
• Stretch in shoulders and chest
• Engagement of glutes and hips

YOU SHOULDN'T FEEL

• Knees collapsing inward; if so, squeeze glutes to draw them back, or use hands to push out
• Arches of feet collapsing; if so, press firmly into toes and balls of feet

Draw ribs in

Pull navel to spine to engage core

Press elbows back to open chest

Reach tailbone down

Press knees backward, keeping them in line with middle toes

2 Lower your hips down into a squat, pressing your knees backward. Tighten your glutes, reach your tailbone down, and press pelvis forward to keep hips under the torso. Keep knees in line with the middle toes. Raise your arms, bend elbows to about 90 degrees, and face your palms forward. Hold the posture, inhaling to reach tailbone down and keep spine neutral, and exhaling to sink deeper into the squat.

ANOTHER VIEW ↻

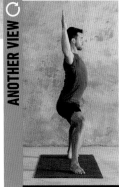

Strive to keep your hips under your torso. Keep your spine as neutral as possible.

HORSE

HIGH LUNGE

No matter your fitness level, try to perform this lunge every single day. This full-body exercise combines hip mobility, core strength, balance, and body control to reduce your risk of injury in the knees, ankles, hips, and spine. This also builds lower-body strength and endurance for improved athletic performance.

TARGET AREAS
• hips • core • spine • lower body

BENEFITS
• Improves hip strength • Relieves stiffness caused by sitting and inactivity • Improves hip mobility • Improves basic balance

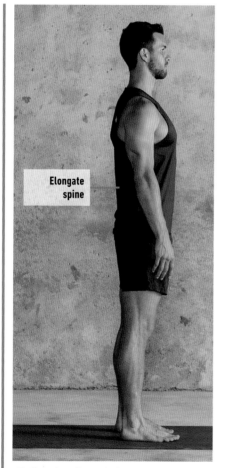

Elongate spine

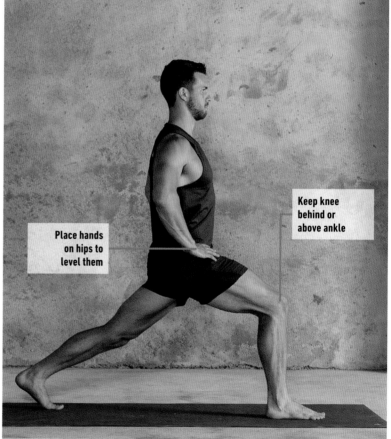

Place hands on hips to level them

Keep knee behind or above ankle

1 Stand at the top of your mat with your feet about 6in (15cm) apart.

2 Take a big step back with your left foot and rise up onto the ball of the left foot. Bend your right knee until the shin is perpendicular to the floor. Press the right heel into the floor to engage your right glutes and hip, and level your hips.

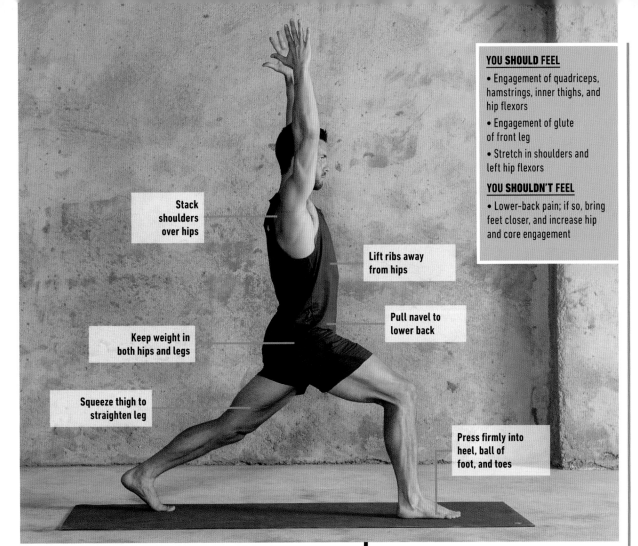

- Engagement of quadriceps, hamstrings, inner thighs, and hip flexors
- Engagement of glute of front leg
- Stretch in shoulders and left hip flexors

YOU SHOULDN'T FEEL
- Lower-back pain; if so, bring feet closer, and increase hip and core engagement

Stack shoulders over hips

Lift ribs away from hips

Keep weight in both hips and legs

Pull navel to lower back

Squeeze thigh to straighten leg

Press firmly into heel, ball of foot, and toes

3 Squeeze your legs toward each other to engage inner thighs and core. Reach your arms straight overhead, keeping the ribs drawn in to prevent chest from splaying open. If front knee passes ankle, shift front foot forward, keeping shin perpendicular to floor. Hold the posture, inhaling as you lengthen the spine and maintain the stance, and exhaling as you sink deeper into the lunge. Repeat on the other side.

NOT THERE YET?

If it's difficult to maintain stability, start with Low lunge (see p58) instead. Bring feet closer toward each other, and rest your back knee on the floor. Once you gain more stability in your legs, you can progress to High lunge.

PRO **TIP**

Use your breathing to work deeper into the pose. After the first 2 or 3 breaths, it is easier to sink deeper while maintaining good technique, so push yourself deeper the longer you hold it.

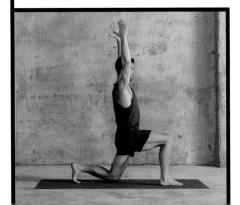

HIGH LUNGE

WARRIOR 1

Warrior 1 is a lunge variation that adds a calf and ankle mobilizing element. It is very effective at improving overall hip mobility, building hip strength, and improving ankle mobility. This makes it great for athletes, especially runners, and anyone who needs to improve lower-body mobility.

TARGET AREAS
• groin • hips • ankles

BENEFITS
• Improves hip mobility and inner thigh strength • Reduces risk of ankle and Achilles tendon injury • Strengthens knees • Reduces lower-back strain

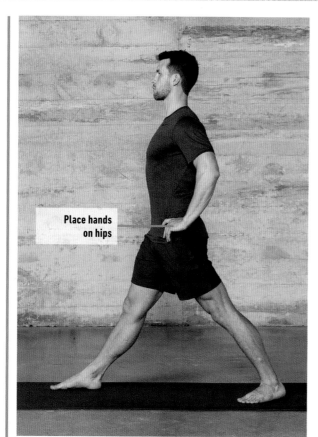

Place hands on hips

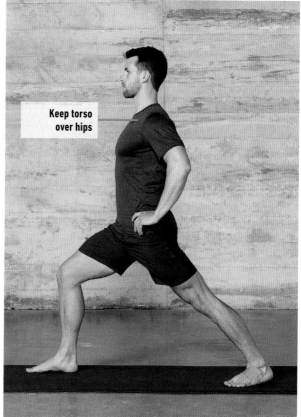

Keep torso over hips

1 From a standing position, take a medium step back with your left foot and place it 4 to 6in (10–15cm) outside your right foot (instead of in a straight line from heel to heel). Point your left foot out at 45 degrees. Straighten legs, and square hips to your right leg.

2 Bend your right knee until your shin is perpendicular to the floor. Keep hips directly under your torso. Squeeze legs toward each other to engage inner thighs, hips, and core. Firmly press through both feet. Keep the back knee locked out.

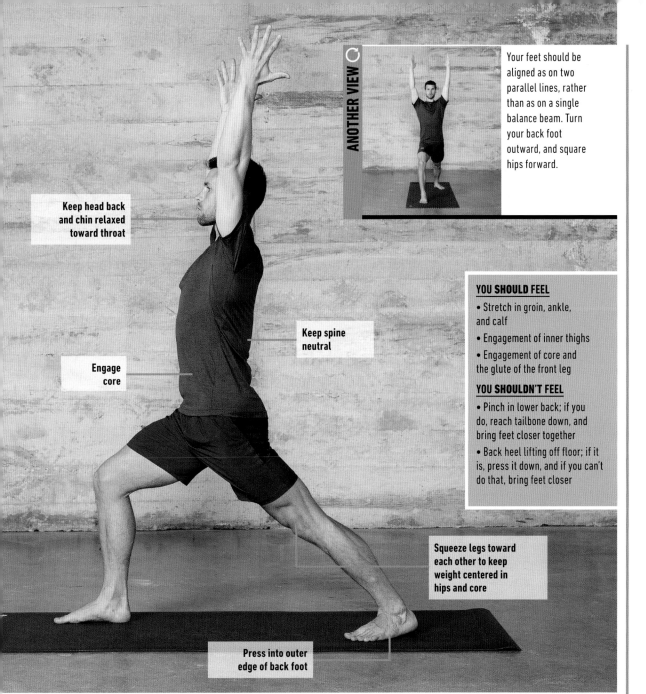

ANOTHER VIEW ⟲

Your feet should be aligned as on two parallel lines, rather than as on a single balance beam. Turn your back foot outward, and square hips forward.

Keep head back and chin relaxed toward throat

Keep spine neutral

Engage core

YOU **SHOULD FEEL**
• Stretch in groin, ankle, and calf
• Engagement of inner thighs
• Engagement of core and the glute of the front leg

YOU **SHOULDN'T FEEL**
• Pinch in lower back; if you do, reach tailbone down, and bring feet closer together
• Back heel lifting off floor; if it is, press it down, and if you can't do that, bring feet closer

Squeeze legs toward each other to keep weight centered in hips and core

Press into outer edge of back foot

3 Lift your arms overhead so your biceps face your ears and palms face each other. Hold the posture, inhaling as you lengthen and get taller, and exhaling as you sink deeper into the lunge. Repeat on the other side.

PRO **TIP**

To square your hips as much as possible, firmly push the front hip toward the floor, and narrow your stance as needed. You may not get them perfectly square, but keep practicing. Focus on feeling the correct stretches in your lower body and making your spine neutral.

HUMBLE WARRIOR

This is a great posture to strengthen and improve shoulder mobility. Add Humble warrior to your daily yoga routine to address shoulder issues, improve your posture, or strengthen your body for more difficult upper-body exercises.

TARGET AREAS
• shoulders • back • hips

BENEFITS
• Improves chest and shoulder mobility • Strengthens upper-back • Balances upper-body muscles • Prevents rotator cuff injury

1 Start in a Warrior 1 stance (see p40), with your left foot back and turned out at 45 degrees, right knee bent, and hips facing forward. Interlace your fingers behind your back, and maintain a firm grip.

PRO **TIP**
This pose is difficult, but the longer you can hold it, the stronger and more mobile your upper back will become. Strive to hold it for 2 or 3 breaths longer than you think you are able.

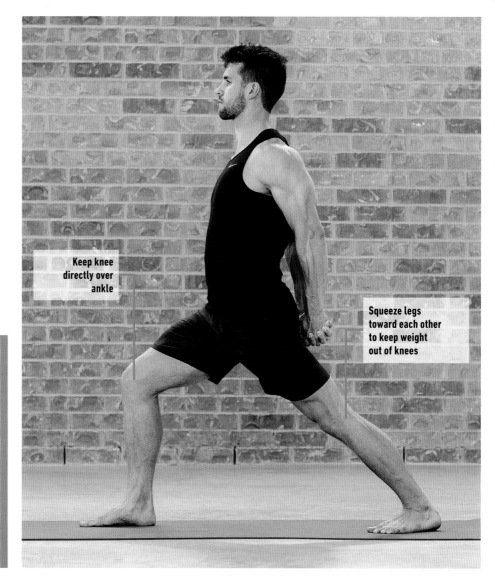

Keep knee directly over ankle

Squeeze legs toward each other to keep weight out of knees

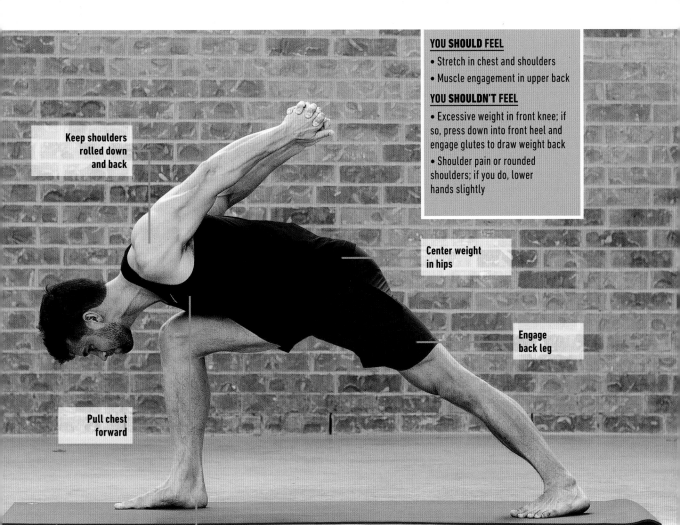

YOU SHOULD FEEL
- Stretch in chest and shoulders
- Muscle engagement in upper back

YOU SHOULDN'T FEEL
- Excessive weight in front knee; if so, press down into front heel and engage glutes to draw weight back
- Shoulder pain or rounded shoulders; if you do, lower hands slightly

Keep shoulders rolled down and back

Center weight in hips

Engage back leg

Pull chest forward

Press down firmly through front heel

2 Inhale deeply to lengthen and get taller, then exhale as you bring your chest forward toward the right thigh. Keep the front of your torso long by maintaining core engagement. Slowly lift your hands away from your back to deepen the shoulder stretch and engage your upper back. Relax your neck and look down at your front foot. Hold the posture, inhaling as you lengthen the spine, and exhaling as you deepen the stretch. Repeat on the other side.

NOT THERE YET?

If your mobility is limited, in step 1, hold a strap behind your back, palms facing toward you. In step 2, lift the strap toward the ceiling, and don't worry about folding as deeply.

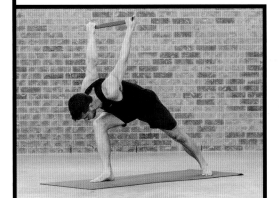

PYRAMID

Pyramid is a very effective pose for increasing mobility in the hamstrings. This makes it ideal for athletes trying to reduce their risk of injury, office workers who spend most of their day sitting, as well as people with chronic lower-back pain. If you want to be able to touch your toes, this is a good pose to work on.

TARGET AREAS
• hamstrings • hips • core

BENEFITS
• Increases hamstring flexibility
• Stretches muscles connected to lower back for lower-back relief
• Decreases risk of hamstring tears and soft-tissue injuries in lower body

1 Start in a Warrior 1 stance (see p40), with your right foot back and turned out at 45 degrees, left knee bent, and hips facing forward.

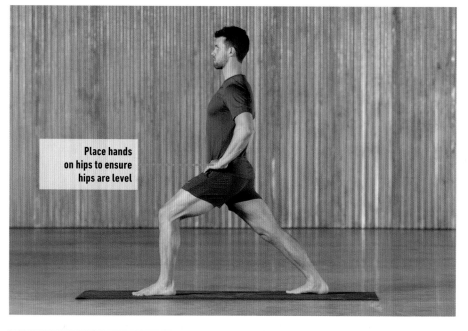

Place hands on hips to ensure hips are level

2 Hinge at the hips and rest fingertips on the floor on either side of front foot. Flatten your back by pulling chest forward and engaging core.

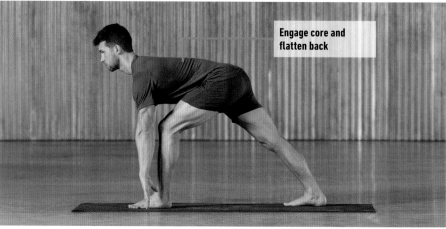

Engage core and flatten back

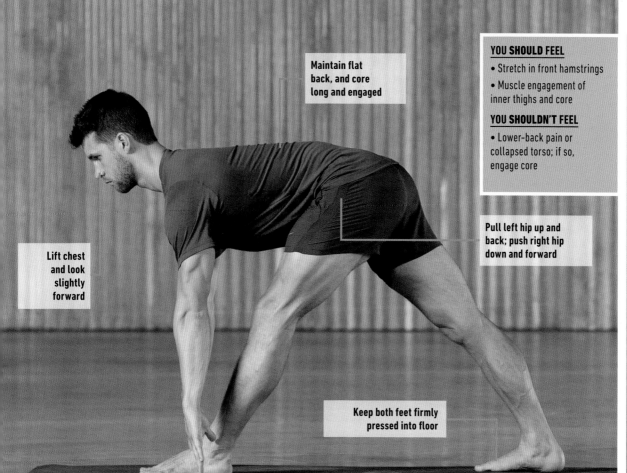

Maintain flat
back, and core
long and engaged

YOU SHOULD FEEL
• Stretch in front hamstrings
• Muscle engagement of inner thighs and core

YOU SHOULDN'T FEEL
• Lower-back pain or collapsed torso; if so, engage core

Pull left hip up and back; push right hip down and forward

Lift chest and look slightly forward

Keep both feet firmly pressed into floor

3 Keeping your back flat and your abs long, slowly straighten your left leg until you feel a stretch in left hamstrings. (It's okay for your left knee to bend as needed.) Squeeze legs toward each other, engaging both quadriceps, and maintain the tension. Hold the posture, inhaling as you lengthen the chest, and exhaling as you deepen the stretch in your hamstrings. Repeat on the other side.

NOT THERE YET?
If your hamstring flexibility is limited or if your spine is rounding, rest your hands on two blocks placed on either side of your front foot.

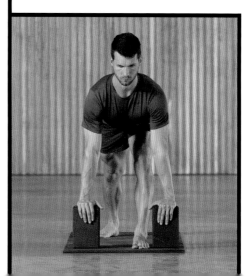

PRO **TIP**
To increase your hamstring strength and mobility, focus on active engagement of the hamstrings in the front leg.

REVOLVED PYRAMID

Use this variation of Pyramid to improve spinal mobility for twists while strengthening the core and improving hip flexibility. This pose is beneficial for athletes, especially triathletes and runners, to prevent back injuries. It also improves potential strength in twisting or swinging movements.

TARGET AREAS
• spine • core • hips

BENEFITS
• Increases spinal mobility for twisting motions • Reduces risk of spinal injury • Improves balance

1 Start in a Warrior 1 stance (see p40), with your left foot back and turned out at 45 degrees, right knee bent, and hips facing forward.

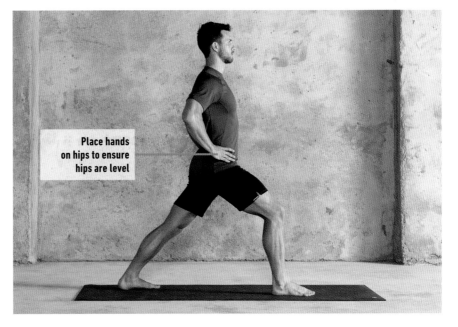

Place hands on hips to ensure hips are level

2 Move into Pyramid (see p44) by hinging at the hips, resting fingertips on the floor, and straightening right leg until you feel a stretch in the right hamstrings. Flatten your back by pulling chest forward. Squeeze legs toward each other. If you cannot keep your back flat while touching the floor, rest left hand on a block.

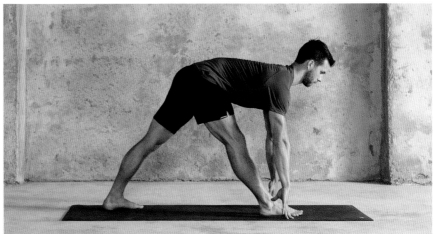

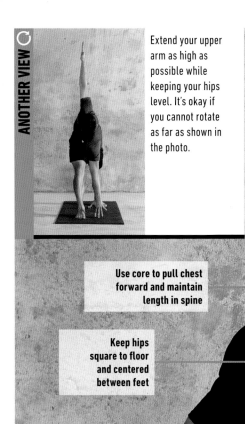

Extend your upper arm as high as possible while keeping your hips level. It's okay if you cannot rotate as far as shown in the photo.

Pull crown of head away from neck and look up at hand

Use core to pull chest forward and maintain length in spine

Keep hips square to floor and centered between feet

YOU SHOULD FEEL
- Stretch in right hamstrings and outer thigh
- Stretch in spine
- Engagement of both legs

YOU SHOULDN'T FEEL
- Discomfort in spine and neck; use core to twist, and maintain maximum length
- Significant weight in front hand; if so, shift weight to hips and core

Keep weight in heels and hips

3 Roll back your right shoulder and extend your right hand toward the ceiling, opening your chest to the right. Use the left fingertips to help maintain balance. Keep hips squared forward, and squeeze legs toward each other. Hold the posture, inhaling as you pull your chest forward and lengthen the spine, and exhaling as you deepen the twist and engage your core. Repeat on the other side.

PRO **TIP**
To challenge your core and legs, try hovering the planted hand above the floor.

REVOLVED PYRAMID

WARRIOR 2

This is an essential lunge posture that builds strength and mobility in the hips, ankles, and core. It's useful for office workers to combat the negative effects of sitting, as well as for athletes to improve hip mobility for more agile change of direction and injury prevention.

TARGET AREAS
• hips • core • ankles

BENEFITS
• Improves groin mobility for lower-back relief • Strengthens hips, knees, and core • Improves lower-body strength and endurance

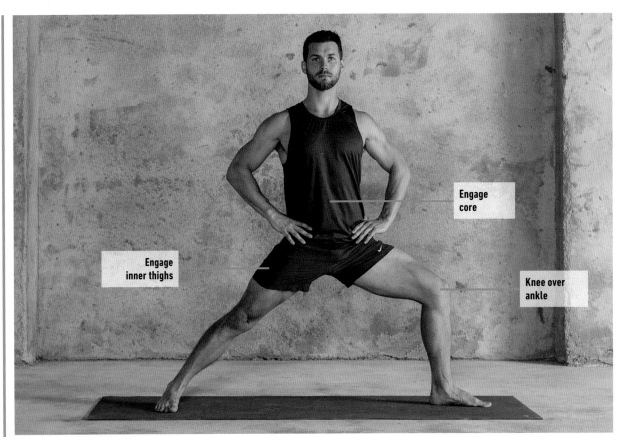

Engage core

Engage inner thighs

Knee over ankle

1 Stand in a wide-legged stance with your feet 4 to 5ft (1.25–1.5m) apart. Turn left foot to face straight outward, and bend the knee until it is directly over your ankle. Place hands on hips to ensure hips are level. Squeeze legs toward each other to engage inner thighs.

PRO **TIP**

To level hips, press the back hip into the front hip and squeeze legs toward each other. Sink deeper into front knee as long as it doesn't cave inward, lower back remains flat, and shoulders stay over hips.

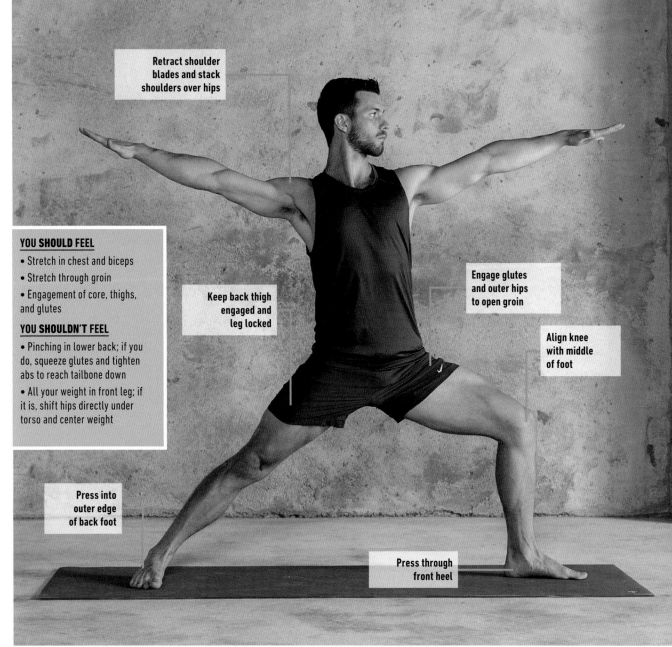

Retract shoulder blades and stack shoulders over hips

YOU SHOULD FEEL
- Stretch in chest and biceps
- Stretch through groin
- Engagement of core, thighs, and glutes

YOU SHOULDN'T FEEL
- Pinching in lower back; if you do, squeeze glutes and tighten abs to reach tailbone down
- All your weight in front leg; if it is, shift hips directly under torso and center weight

Keep back thigh engaged and leg locked

Engage glutes and outer hips to open groin

Align knee with middle of foot

Press into outer edge of back foot

Press through front heel

2 Keeping your torso over your hips, extend your arms to the sides, palms facing down, and press the fingertips of your opposite hands away from one another. Turn your head to gaze down your left arm. Lift ribs away from hips, and maintain tension in legs. Hold the posture, inhaling as you lengthen the spine and grow taller, and exhaling as you sink the hips deeper and engage core. Repeat on the other side.

REVERSE WARRIOR

This posture takes Warrior 2 a step further with a backward bend to stretch your shoulders and back. It is a great movement for desk workers who spend much of their day with their arms at their sides, and for athletes who want to improve shoulder mobility and speed upper-body recovery.

TARGET AREAS
• shoulders • upper back • hips

BENEFITS
• Stretches shoulders and improves upper-body mobility • Reduces risk of rotator cuff injury • Strengthens upper back and neck • Builds lower-body endurance

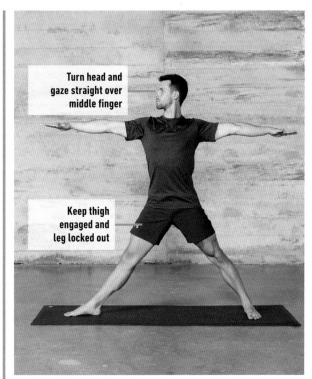

Turn head and gaze straight over middle finger

Keep thigh engaged and leg locked out

1 Stand in a wide-legged stance with your feet 4 to 5ft (1.25–1.5m) apart, and toes turned slightly in. Extend your arms outward, parallel to the floor with your palms facing down. Turn right foot out, nearly perpendicular to the left. Square hips forward, keeping torso over hips.

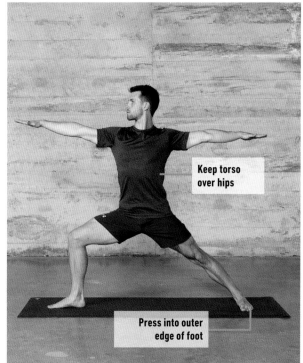

Keep torso over hips

Press into outer edge of foot

2 Sink into Warrior 2 (see p48) by bending your right knee until it is over your ankle. Squeeze legs toward one another to engage inner thighs. If you cannot maintain a neutral spine, bring feet closer together. If your knee moves past your ankle, widen your stance.

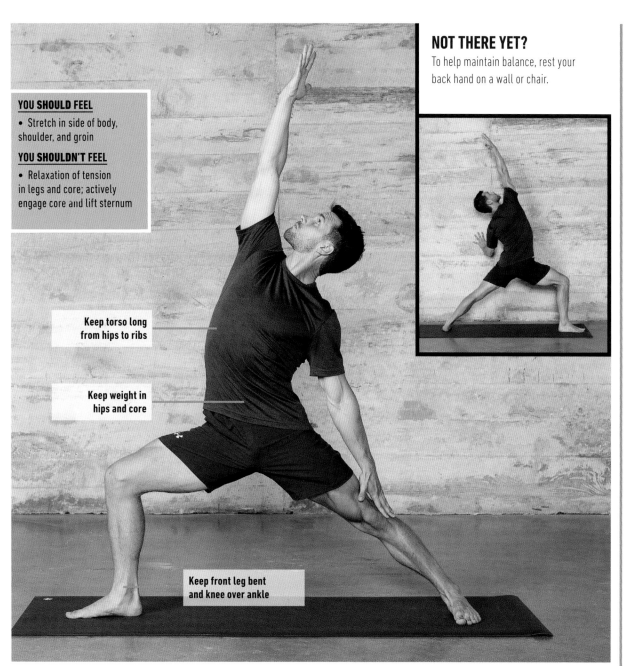

YOU SHOULD FEEL
• Stretch in side of body, shoulder, and groin

YOU SHOULDN'T FEEL
• Relaxation of tension in legs and core; actively engage core and lift sternum

Keep torso long from hips to ribs

Keep weight in hips and core

Keep front leg bent and knee over ankle

3 Maintaining tension in your legs, reach your right arm up toward the ceiling with palm facing backward. Bend backward and rest your left hand lightly on the back leg. Hold the posture, inhaling to lengthen your body, and exhaling to increase the bend and go deeper. Repeat on the other side.

PRO **TIP**
Pretend you're pulling your upper arm out of the socket to reach it as high as possible. Then lean back.

REVERSE WARRIOR

SIDE ANGLE

This side stretch and lunge strengthens your core, hips, and back, while making your spine, shoulders, and hips more mobile. It's useful for improving your posture, increasing power and range of motion for twisting or swinging motions, and helping prevent back pain and injury by strengthening the entire core.

TARGET AREAS
• core • spine • hips • shoulders

BENEFITS
• Stretches chest muscles to improve posture • Strengthens middle back, spine, hips, and knees • Improves spinal mobility

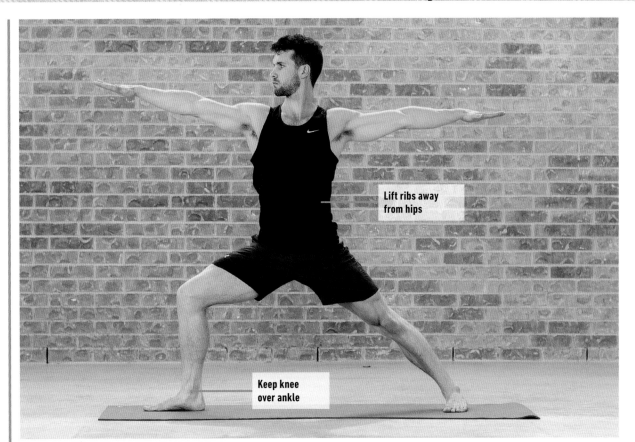

Lift ribs away from hips

Keep knee over ankle

1 Start in Warrior 2 (see p48) with your feet 4 to 5ft (1.25–1.5m) apart, your right foot perpendicular to the left, and front knee bent directly over the ankle. Extend arms outward, parallel to the floor and palms facing down. Square hips to the middle.

PRO **TIP**

To challenge your core and get a deeper stretch, firmly engage the muscles on the exposed side of your body, drawing ribs toward your core to firmly engage obliques and strengthen core.

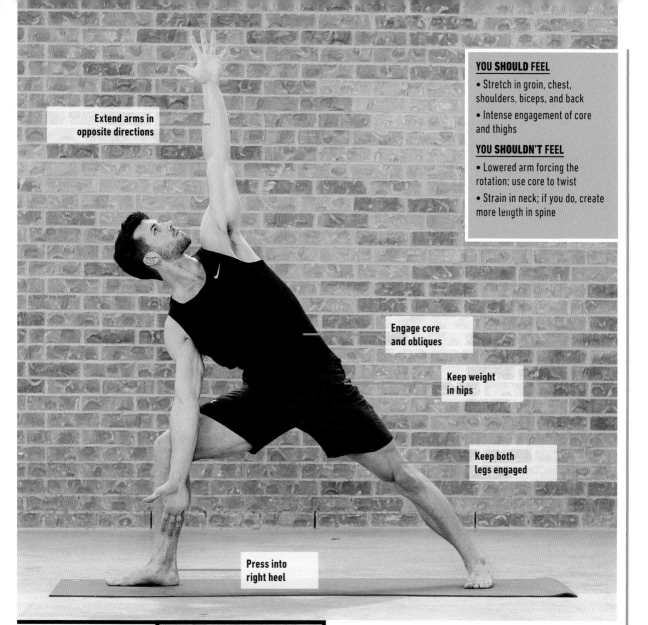

Extend arms in opposite directions

YOU SHOULD FEEL
• Stretch in groin, chest, shoulders, biceps, and back
• Intense engagement of core and thighs

YOU SHOULDN'T FEEL
• Lowered arm forcing the rotation; use core to twist
• Strain in neck; if you do, create more length in spine

Engage core and obliques

Keep weight in hips

Keep both legs engaged

Press into right heel

NOT THERE YET?

To help maintain balance and stability, rest your hand on a block placed just inside the front foot.

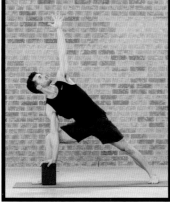

2 Bend at the waist to move the torso over your bent leg. Reach your left arm toward the ceiling, palm facing forward, and extend right arm toward the ground. Tighten the left side of your body, lengthen your torso, and use your core to roll back the top shoulder and open chest. Turn your head to look up at hand. Hold the posture, inhaling as you lengthen the torso, and exhaling as you deepen the twist. Repeat on the other side.

TRIANGLE

This pose builds strength and mobility in your lower body, which helps relieve lower-back discomfort for those who spend a lot of time in a seated position. Triangle is great for martial artists to improve mobility for kicks, and is great for athletes to reduce the risk of soft-tissue injury in the legs and hips.

TARGET AREAS
• hips • inner thighs • core • ankles

BENEFITS
• Increases hip mobility • Relieves lower-back pain caused by sitting and inactivity • Relieves tension in knees • Prevents soft-tissue injury in hips and thighs

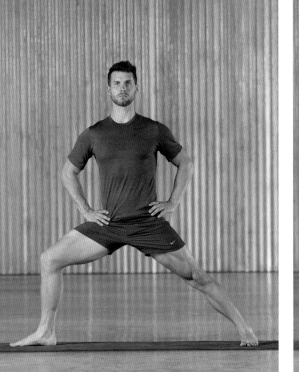

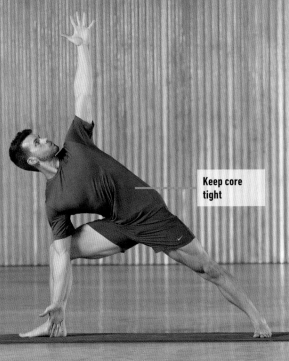

Keep core tight

1 Stand with your feet slightly wider than shoulder-width apart, toes turned slightly in. Turn your right foot outward, perpendicular to the left foot. Place hands on hips to ensure hips are level. Keeping your hips directly under the shoulders and your spine neutral, bend the right knee until it is directly over your ankle.

2 Bend from the waist to move the torso over your bent leg. Reach your left arm toward the ceiling, palm facing forward, and extend your right arm to the floor. Tighten the left side of your body, lengthen your torso, and use your core to roll back the top shoulder and open up the chest. Turn your head to look up at the raised hand.

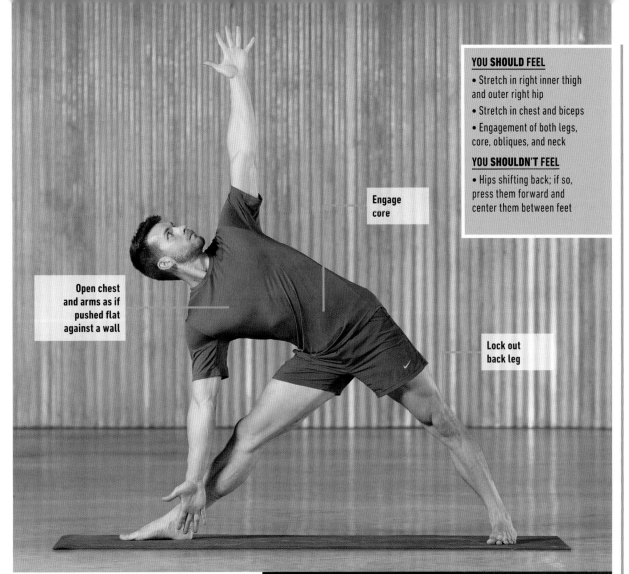

YOU SHOULD FEEL
• Stretch in right inner thigh and outer right hip
• Stretch in chest and biceps
• Engagement of both legs, core, obliques, and neck

YOU SHOULDN'T FEEL
• Hips shifting back; if so, press them forward and center them between feet

Engage core

Open chest and arms as if pushed flat against a wall

Lock out back leg

3 Press through your right heel and slowly straighten the right leg until you feel a stretch in the inner thighs. Press your right hip into your left hip to offset the hips and deepen the inner-thigh stretch. Extend arms as much as possible to stretch the chest and arms. Hold the posture, inhaling as you lengthen the torso and pull your shoulders away from your hips, and exhaling as you deepen the stretch in your inner thighs and tighten your core. Repeat on the other side.

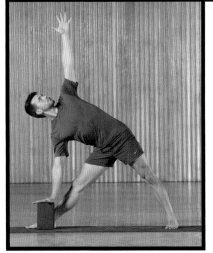

NOT THERE YET?
If you are not quite flexible enough, rest your hand on a block placed inside your front foot. You can also slightly bend your knee as long as you feel the stretch.

TRIANGLE

55

CAT-COW

This slow movement from an arched to rounded spine is one of the best exercises you can do for your back, whether you are an athlete warming up or a non-athlete recovering from a back injury. Use this exercise to mobilize your spine, release kinks or stiffness in your back, and prepare for exercise.

TARGET AREAS
• spine • back • chest

BENEFITS
• Relieves spinal stiffness and pain
• Prevents spinal injury • Improves spinal mobility • Stretches shoulders and back

1 Start on all fours with shoulders over wrists and hips over knees. (Toes can be tucked or untucked.) Position knees and ankles parallel to each other, hip-width apart. Form an L-shape with your index fingers and thumbs.

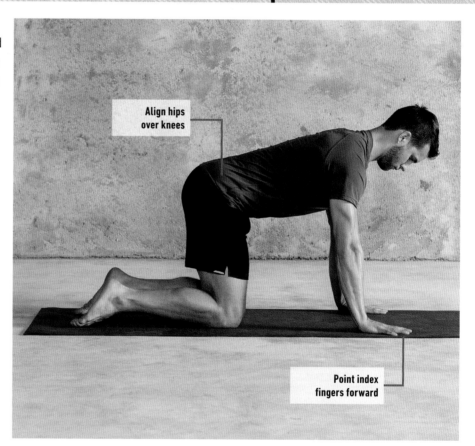

Align hips over knees

Point index fingers forward

PRO **TIP**
Lightly squeeze legs toward one another to keep your core engaged and protect the spine.

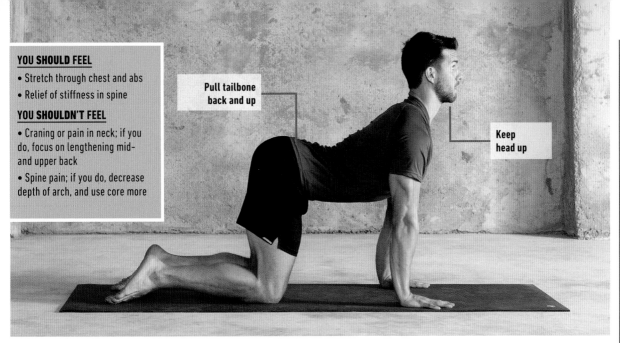

YOU SHOULD FEEL

• Stretch through chest and abs
• Relief of stiffness in spine

YOU SHOULDN'T FEEL

• Craning or pain in neck; if you do, focus on lengthening mid- and upper back
• Spine pain; if you do, decrease depth of arch, and use core more

Pull tailbone back and up

Keep head up

2 Cow: Inhale as you arch your spine, pulling your chest forward and lifting your tailbone toward the ceiling.

Lengthen the front side of your torso, and maintain length in your mid- and upper spine.

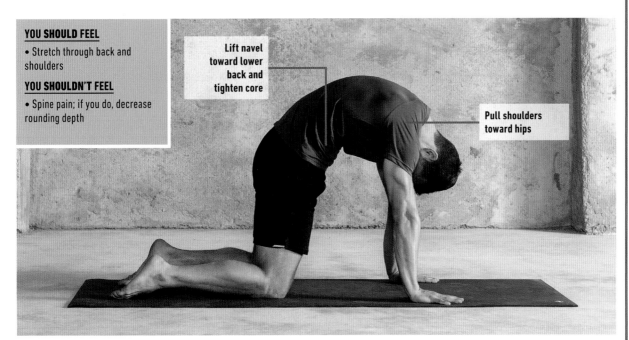

YOU SHOULD FEEL

• Stretch through back and shoulders

YOU SHOULDN'T FEEL

• Spine pain; if you do, decrease rounding depth

Lift navel toward lower back and tighten core

Pull shoulders toward hips

3 Cat: Exhale as you round your spine, pulling your forehead toward your hips. Press down through your hands to lift the upper back toward the ceiling. Tuck your chin to your chest. This is one rep.

Continue to alternate slowly from Cat to Cow, inhaling as you move into the full extension of Cow, and exhaling as you move into the full flexion of Cat. Lengthen each breath as much as possible.

LOW LUNGE

This posture is an essential pillar of a strong lower body. It strengthens your hips, glutes, thighs, and core, improves your hip mobility, and prevents injury in your knees, back, and hips. Low lunge is very important for people who sit often, as well as athletes interested in building power and preventing injury.

TARGET AREAS
• hips • core

BENEFITS
• Improves hip mobility to reduce risk of injury • Builds foundational hip strength and stability

1 Start on all fours with shoulders over wrists and hips over knees. (Toes can be tucked or untucked.) Position knees and ankles parallel to each other, hip-width apart.

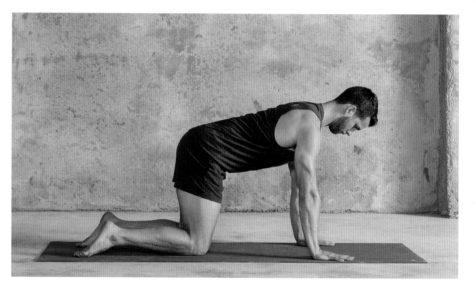

2 Step your right foot up between your hands, bending your right knee to 90 degrees with the knee above the ankle. Let hips sink slightly forward. Press down through the right foot to shift weight into your right hip.

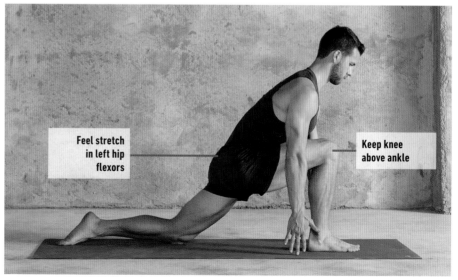

Feel stretch in left hip flexors

Keep knee above ankle

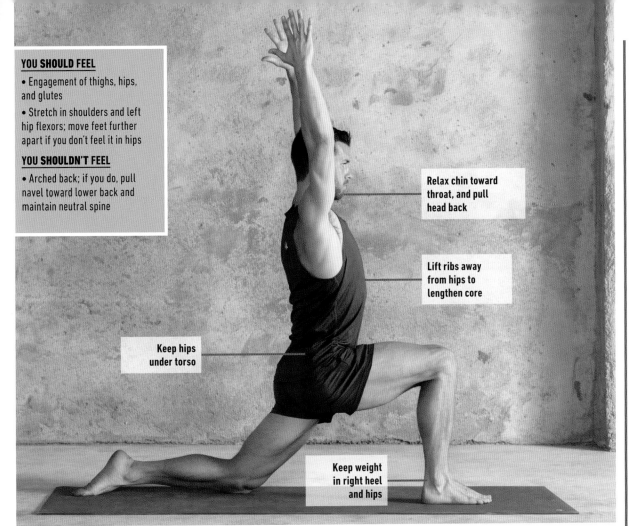

Relax chin toward throat, and pull head back

Lift ribs away from hips to lengthen core

Keep hips under torso

Keep weight in right heel and hips

NOT THERE YET?

If it is difficult to maintain balance, rest one hand on a wall or chair.

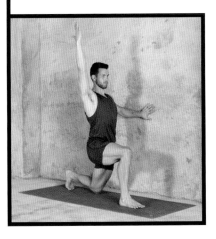

3 Tuck your back toes, engage both thighs, and lift your arms overhead, palms facing each other. Position torso directly over hips. Lightly squeeze inner thighs toward each other. Continue to press down through the right foot. Engage your core and draw ribs in to prevent chest from splaying open. Hold the posture, inhaling as you lift your ribs away from hips, and exhaling as you deepen the hip stretch. Repeat on the other side.

PRO **TIP**

To properly distribute your weight, lift your back knee a few inches off the floor, and notice how your weight shifts into the hip of the front leg. Lower your knee to the floor while maintaining that same level of engagement in the front hip.

RUNNER'S LUNGE

This posture is an excellent lunge for building strength and endurance in the lower body, while also requiring minimal flexibility. As the name suggests, it's perfect for runners to help correct muscle imbalances caused by the repetitive stride motion.

TARGET AREAS
• hips • core • glutes • thighs

BENEFITS
• Improves endurance, muscle activation, and strength in glutes, hips, and thighs • Relieves pressure on knees and reduces risk of injury • Improves hip mobility

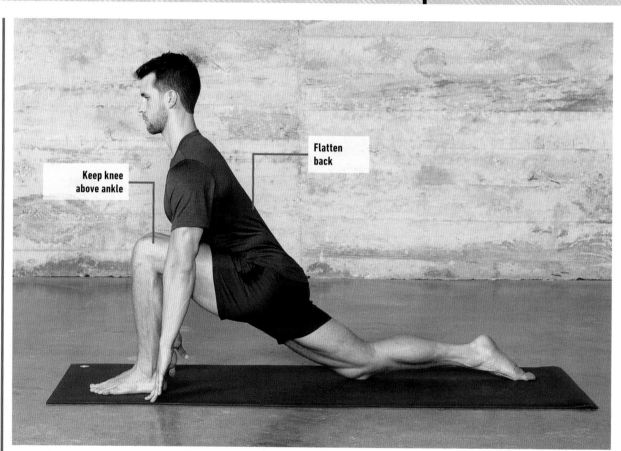

Keep knee above ankle

Flatten back

1 Start on all fours, then step your left foot up between your hands into a Low lunge stance (see p58). Bend your left knee to 90 degrees with the knee above the ankle. Slide right leg back until you feel a stretch in your hips. Rest fingertips on the floor.

PRO **TIP**
To challenge your core and balance, hover your hands above the floor, intensifying core and hip engagement.

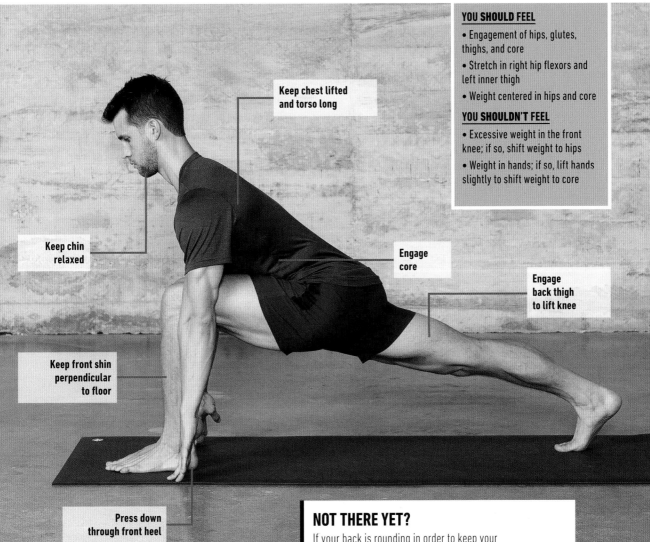

YOU SHOULD FEEL
- Engagement of hips, glutes, thighs, and core
- Stretch in right hip flexors and left inner thigh
- Weight centered in hips and core

YOU SHOULDN'T FEEL
- Excessive weight in the front knee; if so, shift weight to hips
- Weight in hands; if so, lift hands slightly to shift weight to core

Keep chest lifted and torso long

Keep chin relaxed

Engage core

Engage back thigh to lift knee

Keep front shin perpendicular to floor

Press down through front heel

2 Tuck your back toes and squeeze your back thigh to lift the knee. Press down firmly through your left heel, keeping your knee directly over your ankle and hips squared forward. Squeeze your inner thighs toward each other. Pull your chest forward and up to form a straight line from back heel to head, using your core to maintain the position. Hold the posture, inhaling as you lengthen the body, and exhaling as you sink deeper. Repeat on the other side.

NOT THERE YET?

If your back is rounding in order to keep your fingertips on the floor, rest your hands on blocks placed on either side of your front foot to help you form a straight, neutral spine.

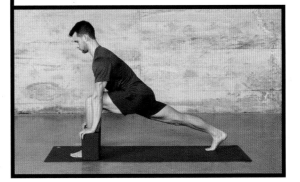

RUNNER'S LUNGE TWIST

Add a rotational element to Runner's lunge to mobilize your spine and build core and lower-body strength. This posture builds strength and stability for hip and spine movements such as twisting and throwing, as well as contributes to quicker and more powerful change of direction. It even improves balance.

TARGET AREAS
• spine • core • hips

BENEFITS
• Strengthens core and spine
• Improves balance and coordination
• Increases spinal mobility for more fluid movement, less stiffness, and reduced risk of injury

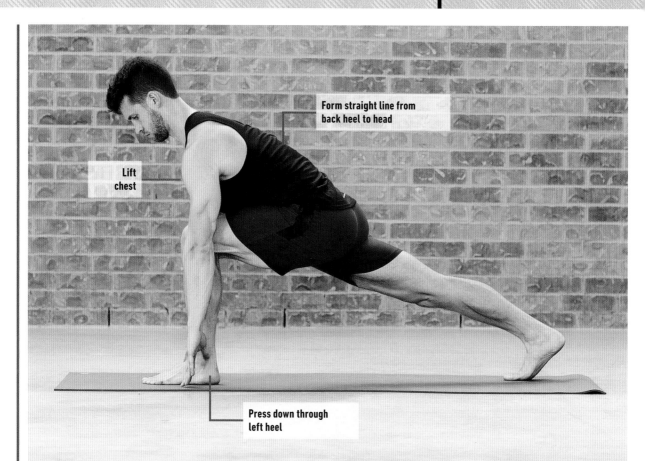

Form straight line from back heel to head

Lift chest

Press down through left heel

1 Start in Runner's lunge (see p60) with your left knee over your ankle and your right leg straight. Place your fingertips on the floor. Squeeze inner thighs toward each other, and pull chest forward and up to form a straight line from back heel to head.

PRO **TIP**

To achieve a deep rotation of the spine, bring the upper arm across your back to rest on the opposite hip, and roll back the top shoulder as much as possible while keeping hips level.

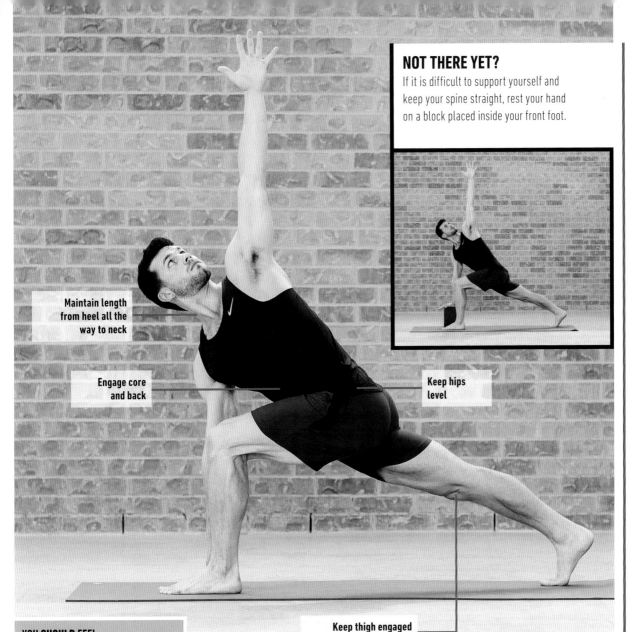

NOT THERE YET?

If it is difficult to support yourself and keep your spine straight, rest your hand on a block placed inside your front foot.

Maintain length from heel all the way to neck

Engage core and back

Keep hips level

Keep thigh engaged and knee lifted

YOU SHOULD FEEL

• Engagement of hips

• Stretch in right hip flexors, middle back, and spine

YOU SHOULDN'T FEEL

• Weight in right hand; if it is, shift weight back into hips

• Hips shifting to side; if so, bring back to middle and reduce rotation

• Neck discomfort; if you do, press crown of head away from shoulders

2 Extend your right arm straight up toward the ceiling. Use your core to roll back the left shoulder and open chest, keeping hips square to the floor. Turn your head to look up at your hand. Hold the posture, inhaling as you lengthen the torso, and exhaling as you deepen the rotation. Repeat on the other side.

HALF SPLIT

Want to touch your toes? This helps. This stretch targets the hamstrings and calves to improve flexibility, reduce soreness, and relieve pressure on the lower back. You can use this to warm up for a workout, relieve soreness the day after a workout, or loosen tight muscles after long periods of sitting.

TARGET AREAS
• hamstrings • calves

BENEFITS
• Promotes quick lower-body recovery • Reduces lower-back pressure or pain caused by hip tightness • Reduces risk of hamstring injury

1 Start in Low lunge (see p58) with your left knee above your ankle and your right knee and foot resting on the floor, toes untucked. Place hands on hips to ensure hips are level.

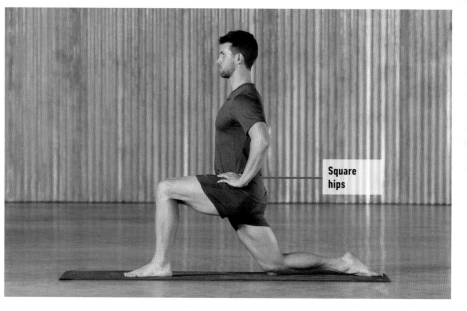

Square hips

2 Hinge forward to rest your fingertips on the floor on either side of your heel. Inch left foot forward 4 to 6in (10–15cm), then shift hips back.

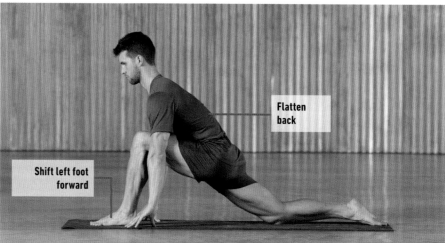

Flatten back

Shift left foot forward

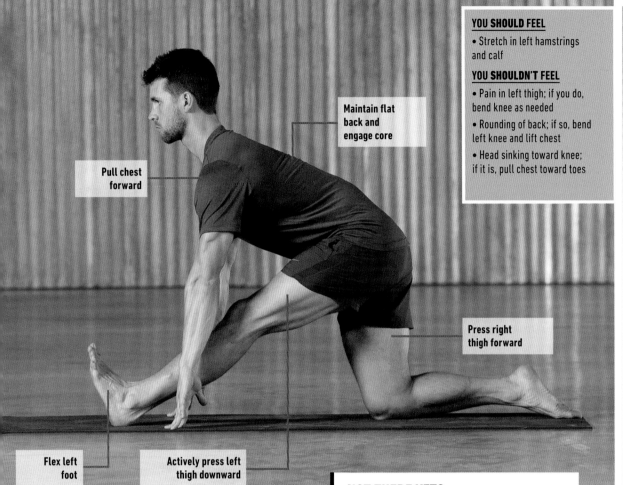

Pull chest forward

Maintain flat back and engage core

YOU SHOULD FEEL
- Stretch in left hamstrings and calf

YOU SHOULDN'T FEEL
- Pain in left thigh; if you do, bend knee as needed
- Rounding of back; if so, bend left knee and lift chest
- Head sinking toward knee; if it is, pull chest toward toes

Press right thigh forward

Flex left foot

Actively press left thigh downward

3 Flex the toes of your left foot toward your shin, and press your left thigh toward the floor until you feel a stretch through left hamstrings. Relax your neck. Hold the posture, inhaling as you lengthen the spine, and exhaling as you deepen the stretch in the hamstrings. Repeat on the other side.

PRO **TIP**

To make the pose more active and improve hamstring mobility, make sure to engage your lower-body muscles. Squeeze the back thigh forward, press front hamstrings downward, and squeeze hips toward each other.

NOT THERE YET?
If you cannot flatten your back with your hands on the floor, rest your hands on blocks placed on either side of your front shin.

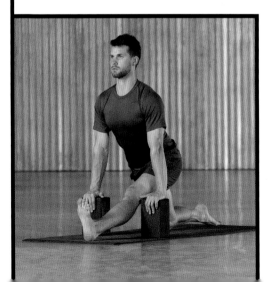

LIZARD

This deep-lunge stretch opens the hips, releases tension in your back, and decreases soreness in the lower body. Lizard helps speed up recovery and reduces the risk of injury in the hips, thighs, knees, and lower back. It also helps reverse the negative effects of prolonged sitting or inactivity.

TARGET AREAS
• hip flexors • inner thighs

BENEFITS
• Relieves hip tension and soreness • Increases hip flexibility for longer strides and deeper lunges • Prevents common soft-tissue hip injuries • Reduces lower-back pressure

1 Start in Plank (see p88) with your shoulders over your wrists and your core engaged. Form a straight line from head to heels.

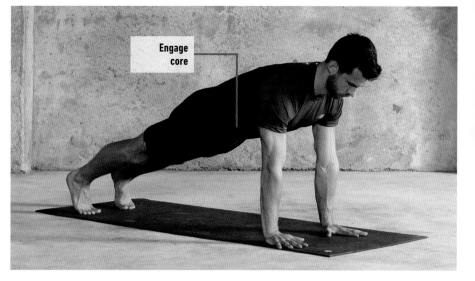

Engage core

2 Step your left foot to the outside of your left hand. Align left knee over the ankle. Keep core engaged and hips level. If this movement from plank is difficult, rest your knees on the floor, then step the foot up.

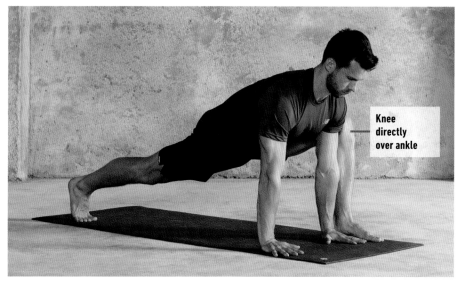

Knee directly over ankle

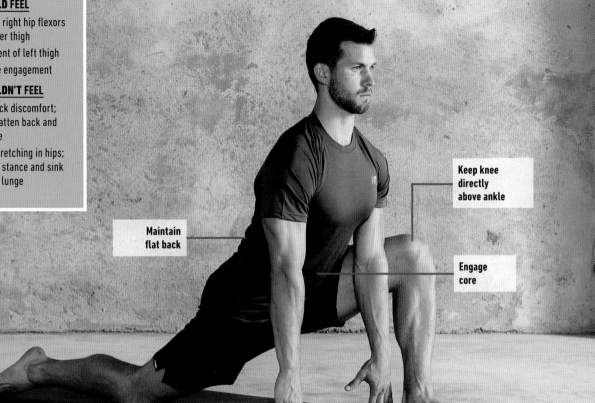

YOU **SHOULD FEEL**
• Stretch in right hip flexors and left inner thigh
• Engagement of left thigh
• Light core engagement

YOU **SHOULDN'T FEEL**
• Lower-back discomfort; if you do, flatten back and engage core
• Lack of stretching in hips; if so, widen stance and sink deeper into lunge

Keep knee directly above ankle

Maintain flat back

Engage core

Lightly rest fingertips on floor

NOT THERE YET?
To help prevent back from rounding, rest hands on a block placed just inside the front foot.

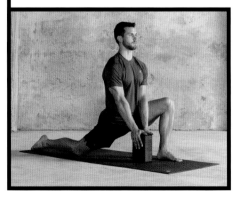

3 Lower your right knee to the floor and untuck your toes. Shift left foot forward and to the left a few inches until you feel a deep stretch in the right hip. Inch your right foot back to extend the right leg as far as you are able. Lift your chest. Maintain a flat or slightly arched back. Hold the posture, inhaling as you lengthen and lift the spine, and exhaling as you sink hips deeper. Repeat on the other side.

PRO **TIP**
Press the top of your back foot into the floor and squeeze the back thigh to increase the intensity of this stretch.

LIZARD

AIRPLANE

This posture increases hamstring strength and mobility, strengthens the core, teaches proper hip engagement, and improves balance. It also helps prevent common soft-tissue injuries in the knees, ankles, and hips. Master this pose to significantly increase the strength potential of your lower body.

TARGET AREAS
• hamstrings • hips • glutes • core

BENEFITS
• Improves lower-body power and muscle engagement • Improves balance • Increases hamstrings mobility for faster recovery, reduced risk of injury, and a stronger spine

1 Stand in the center of your mat and step your left foot back 2 to 3ft (0.5–1m). Rise onto the ball of the left foot and bend your right knee into a shallow lunge. Keep hips and feet facing forward. Lengthen torso and keep chest upright. Place hands on hips to ensure hips are level.

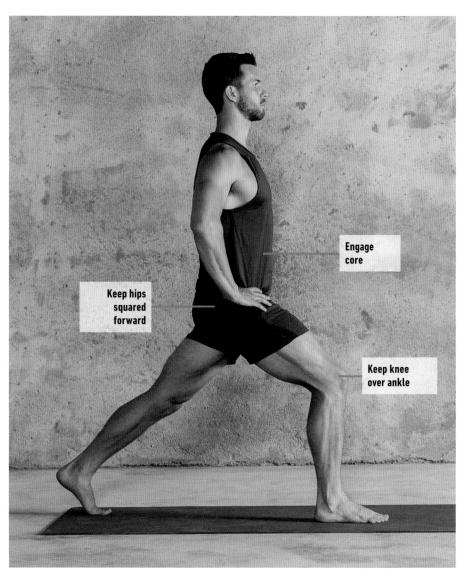

Engage core

Keep hips squared forward

Keep knee over ankle

PRO **TIP**
Square your hips before you rise off the floor. You shouldn't have to readjust later on.

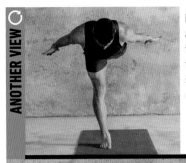

Let your left hip relax down and squeeze your right glute to square your hips to the floor. Your entire right leg should be engaged for the duration of this posture.

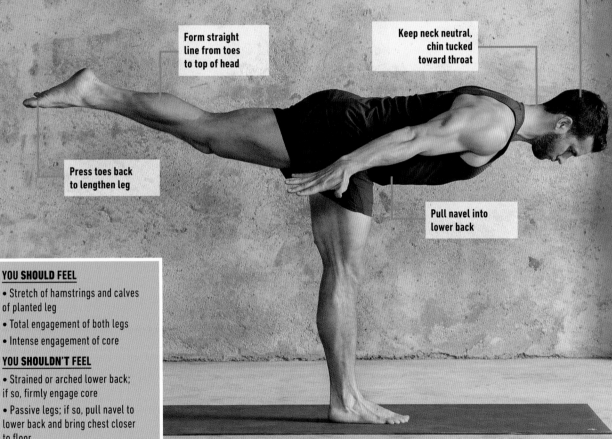

Press crown of head forward to lengthen

Keep neck neutral, chin tucked toward throat

Form straight line from toes to top of head

Press toes back to lengthen leg

Pull navel into lower back

YOU SHOULD FEEL
• Stretch of hamstrings and calves of planted leg
• Total engagement of both legs
• Intense engagement of core

YOU SHOULDN'T FEEL
• Strained or arched lower back; if so, firmly engage core
• Passive legs; if so, pull navel to lower back and bring chest closer to floor

2 Inhale to prepare to lift off your back leg, then exhale as you press down into your right heel and lift the left leg. Hinge at the hips and bring your torso parallel to the floor. (Bend your knee if necessary.) Point the toes of your left foot, engage your entire left leg, and reach your left leg back as far as possible. Firmly engage glutes and core.

Press the crown of head forward to lengthen torso. Extend arms back along your sides, palms facing the floor. Hold the posture, inhaling as you lengthen the body, and exhaling as you squeeze core, hips, and thighs. Repeat on other side.

WARRIOR 3

Get ready to work your entire body. This challenging balance posture develops strength and mobility in your lower body, core, and shoulders. You will hold it for much less time than other yoga postures, but that just means you need to give it your all when you do it. If it's too difficult, master Airplane first.

1 Stand in the middle of your mat and step your left foot back 2 to 3ft (0.5–1m). Rise onto the ball of your left foot and bend your right knee into a shallow lunge. Keep hips and feet facing forward. Lengthen torso and keep chest upright. Raise your arms overhead, press palms together, and interlace fingers with index fingers extended.

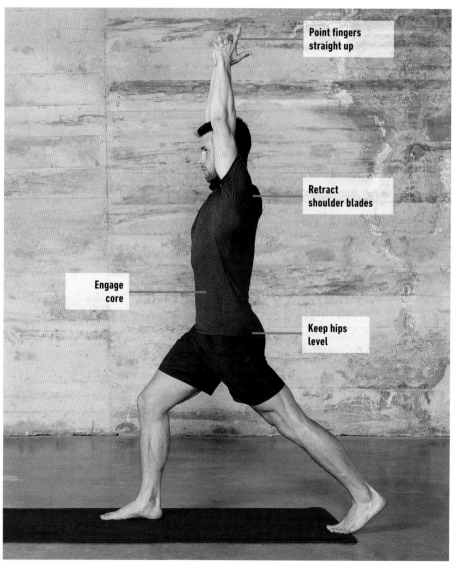

Point fingers straight up

Retract shoulder blades

Engage core

Keep hips level

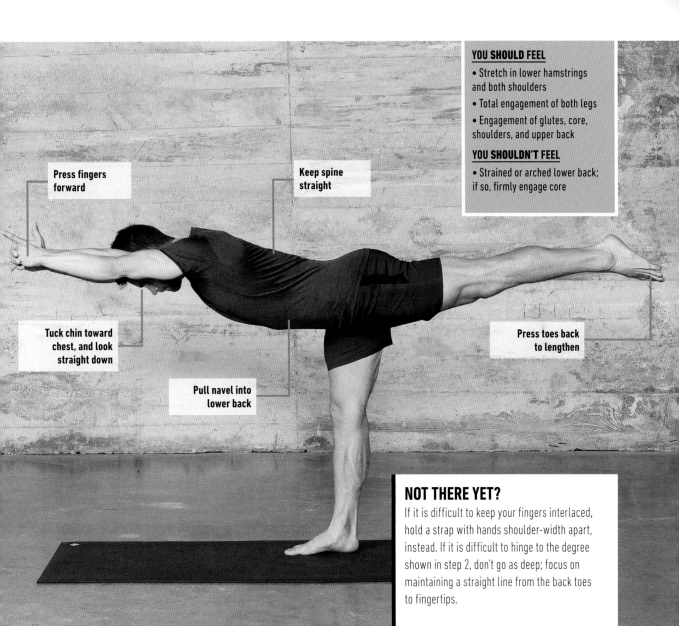

Press fingers forward

Keep spine straight

Tuck chin toward chest, and look straight down

Press toes back to lengthen

Pull navel into lower back

NOT THERE YET?
If it is difficult to keep your fingers interlaced, hold a strap with hands shoulder-width apart, instead. If it is difficult to hinge to the degree shown in step 2, don't go as deep; focus on maintaining a straight line from the back toes to fingertips.

2 Inhale as you lengthen your body, then exhale as you press down through the right foot and lift left leg. Hinge at the hips until your torso is parallel to the floor, and straighten your left leg until you feel a stretch through left hamstrings. (You don't have to lock your leg.) Firmly engage glutes and core to keep torso and left leg in a straight line. Make body as long as possible by pressing fingertips and toes away from each other. Hold the posture, inhaling as you lengthen the spine, and exhaling as you tighten your core. Repeat on the other side.

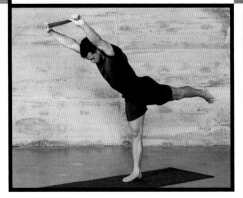

EAGLE

This pose strengthens the hips and glutes, improves balance, and stretches the upper back and shoulders. Eagle helps keep your shoulders healthy and prevent rotator cuff injury. It is useful to practice the leg and arm positions separately before putting them together.

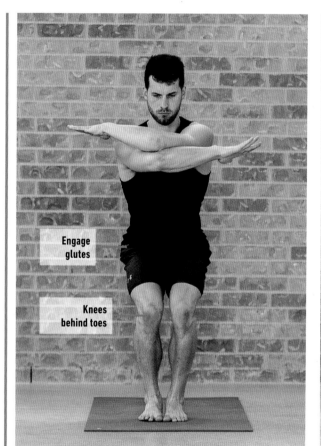

Engage glutes

Knees behind toes

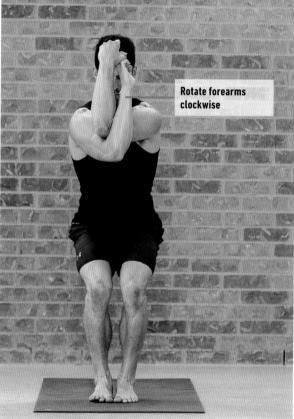

Rotate forearms clockwise

1 Stand in Mountain pose (see p20) with big toes touching and heels about 1in (2.5cm) apart. Squat hips down and back while squeezing inner thighs toward each other. Reach your right arm under your left arm, stacking elbows on top of each other.

2 Lift your forearms upward, and link your fingers together. Firmly maintain the squat position. If you can't link your fingers, just press arms toward each other.

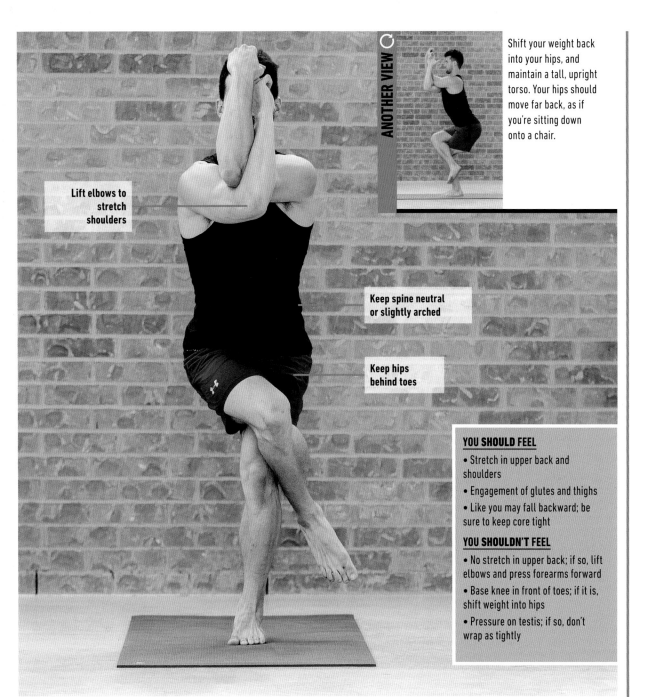

Shift your weight back into your hips, and maintain a tall, upright torso. Your hips should move far back, as if you're sitting down onto a chair.

Lift elbows to stretch shoulders

Keep spine neutral or slightly arched

Keep hips behind toes

YOU SHOULD FEEL

- Stretch in upper back and shoulders
- Engagement of glutes and thighs
- Like you may fall backward; be sure to keep core tight

YOU SHOULDN'T FEEL

- No stretch in upper back; if so, lift elbows and press forearms forward
- Base knee in front of toes; if it is, shift weight into hips
- Pressure on testis; if so, don't wrap as tightly

PRO **TIP**

If you aren't flexible enough yet, grab your opposite shoulder blades (like a hug) and stretch them apart.

3 Slowly lift your right leg and wrap it around your left thigh. Tightly squeeze thighs together and keep hips level. Lift ribs away from your hips and lean backward, as much as you are able, to engage your hips and core. Hold the posture, inhaling as you lift your chest, and exhaling as you sit deeper. Repeat on the other side.

TREE

This is one of the most basic balancing poses in yoga. It is extremely good at building strength and balance. Tree increases hip mobility and strength in the lower body, prevents injury in the knees, and improves overall balance. It even opens your chest and improves your posture. There is no reason not to love it!

TARGET AREAS
• hips • core

BENEFITS
• Strengthens hips and glutes
• Improves balance • Strengthens and prevents lower-back, knee, and ankle injury • Improves hip stability and neutralizes alignment

1 Stand in Mountain pose (see p20) with big toes touching and heels about 1in (2.5cm) apart. Lift your right leg and press your foot into the left thigh or shin (but avoid the knee), toes pointed down. You can use your hand to help position the foot securely on your leg.

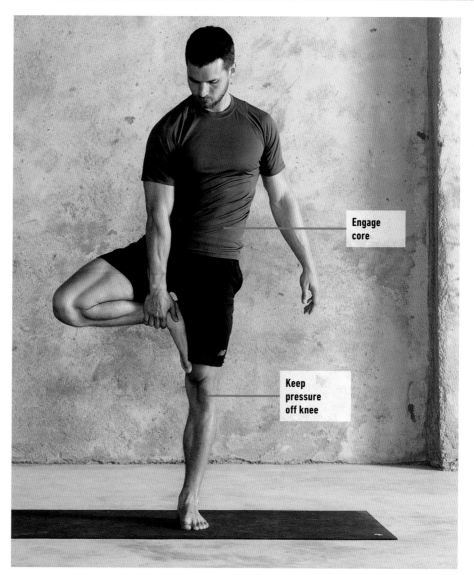

Engage core

Keep pressure off knee

PRO **TIP**
This is a fantastic posture for activating your core and hips. Squeeze your glutes as tightly as possible, and work on getting the lifted knee to face directly to the outside.

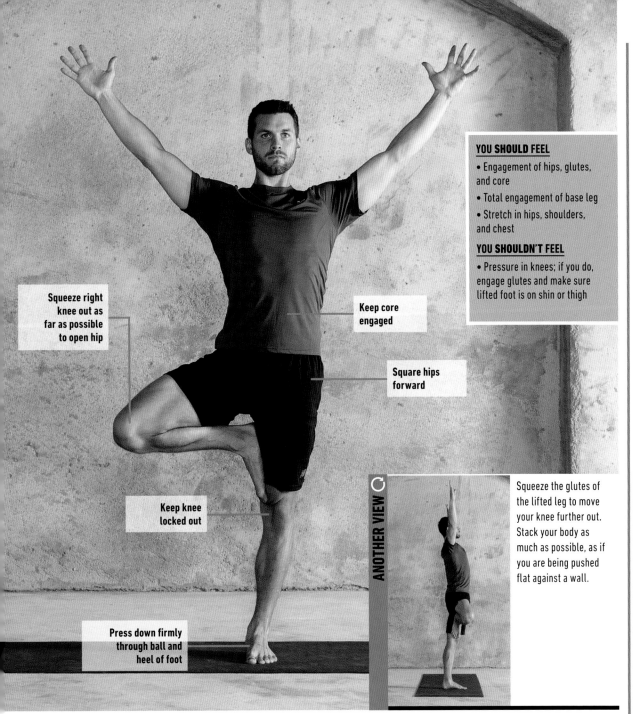

Squeeze right knee out as far as possible to open hip

Keep core engaged

Square hips forward

Keep knee locked out

Press down firmly through ball and heel of foot

YOU SHOULD FEEL
- Engagement of hips, glutes, and core
- Total engagement of base leg
- Stretch in hips, shoulders, and chest

YOU SHOULDN'T FEEL
- Pressure in knees; if you do, engage glutes and make sure lifted foot is on shin or thigh

ANOTHER VIEW ↻

Squeeze the glutes of the lifted leg to move your knee further out. Stack your body as much as possible, as if you are being pushed flat against a wall.

2 Extend your arms overhead in a V-shape, palms facing forward. Squeeze your right glute to rotate right hip outward and open the hip. Keep hips facing forward. Reach tailbone toward the floor to engage core and lengthen lower back. Hold the posture, inhaling as you lengthen the torso, and exhaling to increase engagement of core, thighs, and hips. Repeat on the other side.

STANDING BOW

This is a great balancing exercise to increase hip mobility, stretch your chest and shoulders, and strengthen the spine. The combination of stretching and strengthening the core is great for endurance athletes. It's also beneficial for anyone who sits often to strengthen the muscles that get weak.

TARGET AREAS
• hips • spine • shoulders

BENEFITS
• Increases hip mobility
• Strengthens spine • Improves balance • Increases lower-body endurance and strength

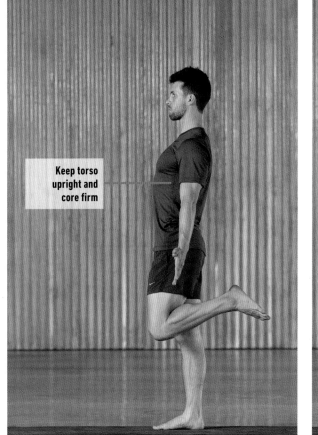

Keep torso upright and core firm

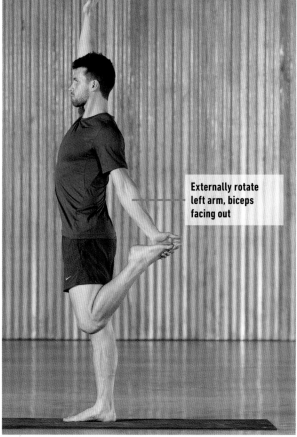

Externally rotate left arm, biceps facing out

1 Stand in Mountain pose (see p20) with big toes touching and heels about 1in (2.5cm) apart. Face your palms forward to open the chest. Lift your left foot, bend the leg behind you, and squeeze leg to pull heel toward glutes.

2 Reach back with your left hand and grasp the inside of your left foot. Extend your right arm straight up. Press into the floor with your right foot. Inhale as you lengthen your body and reach fingertips higher.

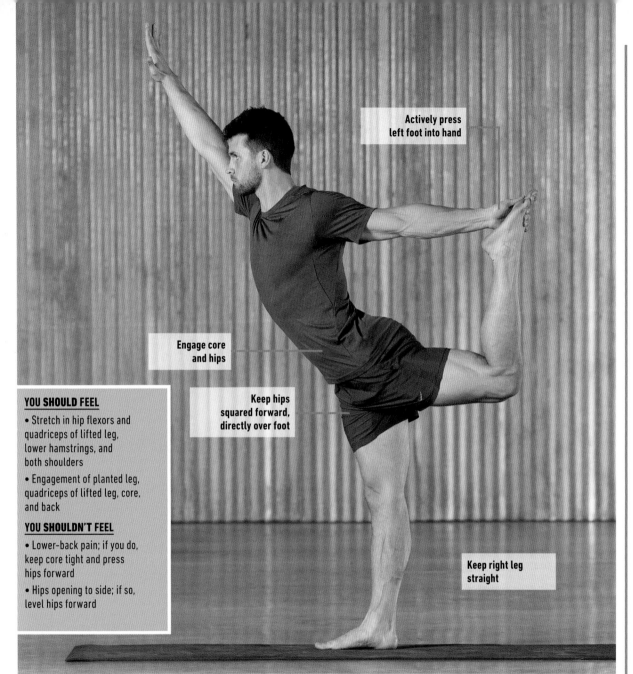

**Actively press
left foot into hand**

**Engage core
and hips**

**Keep hips
squared forward,
directly over foot**

**Keep right leg
straight**

YOU SHOULD FEEL
• Stretch in hip flexors and
quadriceps of lifted leg,
lower hamstrings, and
both shoulders
• Engagement of planted leg,
quadriceps of lifted leg, core,
and back

YOU SHOULDN'T FEEL
• Lower-back pain; if you do,
keep core tight and press
hips forward
• Hips opening to side; if so,
level hips forward

3 Exhale as you press your left foot firmly into your left
hand, using this force to stretch the left hip flexors.
Hinge at the hips to bring torso forward and down as you
press lifted leg back and up. Keep right arm extended.
Engage core, and reach tailbone back to lengthen the lower
back. Hold the posture, inhaling as you lengthen the torso,
and exhaling as you press deeper. Repeat on the other side.

PRO **TIP**
To build active hip mobility, focus on
engaging the hip flexors in your lifted
leg. This builds active flexibility, which
leads to more functional strength and
decreased risk of injury.

STANDING FINGER-TO-TOE

This balancing posture provides a deep hamstring and calf stretch, while improving strength and mobility in your core and hips. It is good for athletes to help prevent common soft-tissue injuries in the lower body, as well as an excellent stretch for runners to correct muscle imbalances.

TARGET AREAS
• hamstrings • calves • hips • core

BENEFITS
• Improves calf, hamstring, and hip mobility • Strengthens and prevents knee injury • Strengthens calves, hips, thighs, and core

1 Stand in Mountain pose (see p20) with big toes touching and heels about 1in (2.5cm) apart. Lift your right foot off the floor and grab your big toe with your right index and middle finger. Keep your arm inside your lifted leg.

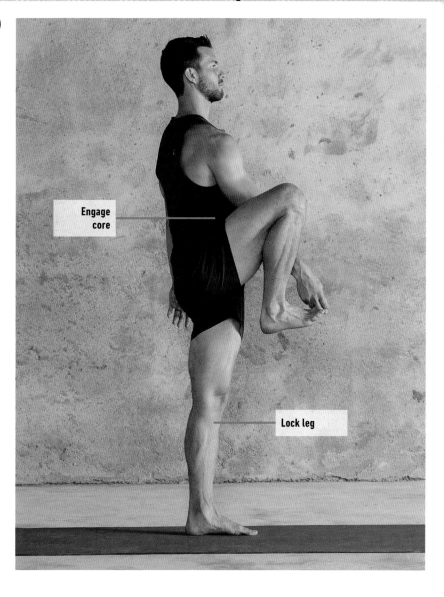

Engage core

Lock leg

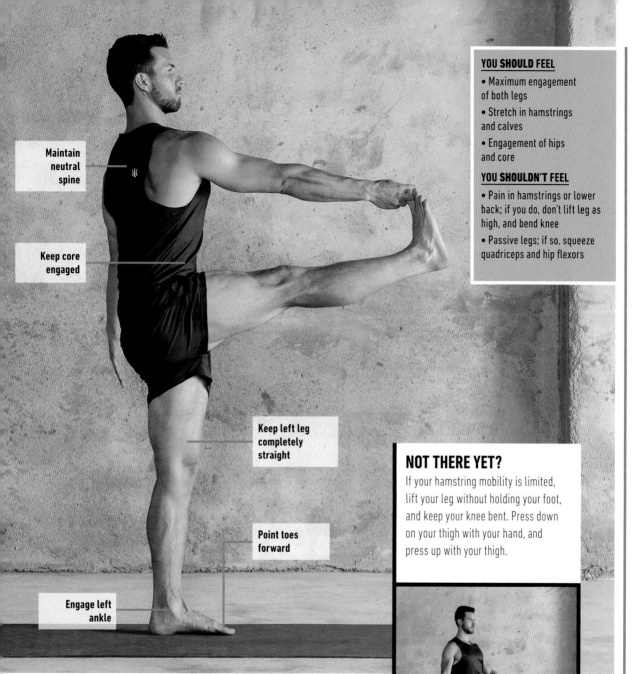

Maintain neutral spine

Keep core engaged

Keep left leg completely straight

Point toes forward

Engage left ankle

YOU SHOULD FEEL

- Maximum engagement of both legs
- Stretch in hamstrings and calves
- Engagement of hips and core

YOU SHOULDN'T FEEL

- Pain in hamstrings or lower back; if you do, don't lift leg as high, and bend knee
- Passive legs; if so, squeeze quadriceps and hip flexors

NOT THERE YET?

If your hamstring mobility is limited, lift your leg without holding your foot, and keep your knee bent. Press down on your thigh with your hand, and press up with your thigh.

2 While keeping your left leg straight and quadriceps fully engaged, slowly straighten the right leg until you feel a stretch in the right hamstrings. Keep chest upright, core engaged, and hips level. Press down firmly through the planted foot to lift hips and stand as tall as possible. Hold the posture, inhaling as you lift and get taller, and exhaling as you press your foot further forward and maintain the lift in your leg. Repeat on the other side.

STANDING FINGER-TO-TOE

BOAT

This very challenging posture works your transverse abdominals—the deep core muscles that keep you upright, help you balance, and enable you to do just about any movement with safe and proper technique. Use this pose to strengthen your core and improve muscle efficiency in full-body movements.

TARGET AREAS
• core • hips • spine

BENEFITS
• Improves balance postures, squats, and backbends • Prevents lower-back pain • Strengthens core • Improves posture • Reduces risk of knee and hip injury

1 Sit on the floor, bend your knees, and place your feet flat on the floor, with your heels 1½ to 2ft (45–60cm) away from your hips. Lightly grip your knees with your hands, sit as upright as possible, and lean back slightly.

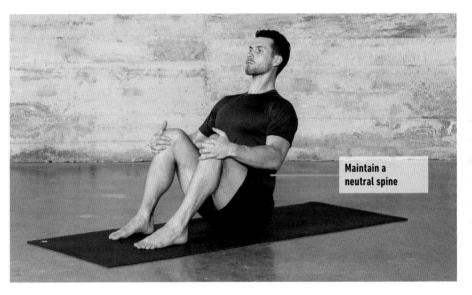

Maintain a neutral spine

2 Keeping your chest lifted and your torso still, squeeze your hip flexors and abdominal muscles toward each other to engage core. Let go of knees, and reach arms forward and up, palms up.

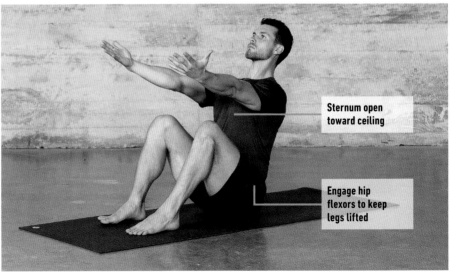

Sternum open toward ceiling

Engage hip flexors to keep legs lifted

Lift knees toward ceiling

Maintain neutral back

Press lower back forward into navel

YOU SHOULD FEEL

• Engagement of core and hip flexors

• Openness in chest

YOU SHOULDN'T FEEL

• Relaxed hip flexors; if so, lift legs higher and lean back a little more

• Lower-back pain; if you do, engage core and hips

• Arched neck; if so, lower chin so neck is neutral

3 Continue to firmly engage your abdominal muscles and hip flexors, and slowly lift feet off the floor and straighten legs. Pull sternum toward the ceiling while keeping spine neutral. Hold the posture, inhaling as you lengthen the spine, and exhaling as you tighten the core.

NOT THERE YET?

If you are unable to extend your legs without your chest caving in, keep legs bent, lightly rest feet on the floor, or keep hands lightly wrapped around knees for support.

PRO **TIP**

While you are still holding your knees, use a mirror to ensure that your chest is lifted and spine is a straight line. When you lift your hands, notice the intense core engagement required to maintain the straight spine.

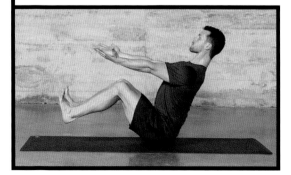

BOAT

BUTTERFLY STRETCH

This groin stretch is beneficial for most men—especially office workers and athletes—because it releases tight hips and improves mobility. Do this stretch both before and after a workout to mobilize your hips and relieve lower-back pressure, or anytime you're feeling tight and want a quick stretch.

TARGET AREAS
• groin • core

BENEFITS
• Stretches groin and increases flexibility • Relieves lower-back pain • Improves mobility for squats, lunges, and other lower-body movements

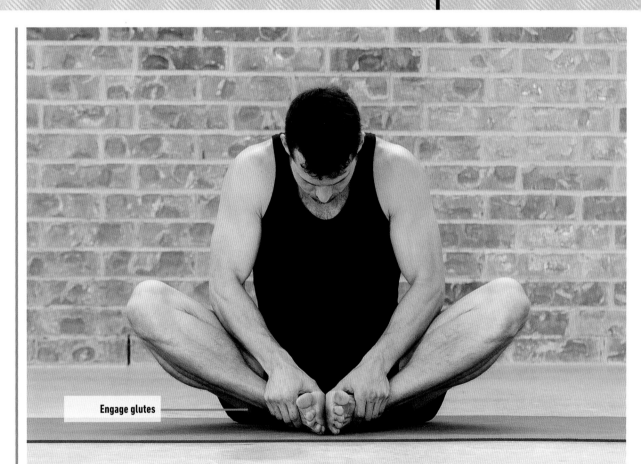

Engage glutes

1 Sit on the floor, place the soles of your feet together, and squeeze your glutes to point the knees out to the sides. Grip both ankles or feet for stability.

PRO **TIP**
If this stretch is too easy, pull heels in closer to your groin. Just be careful not to strain your knees.

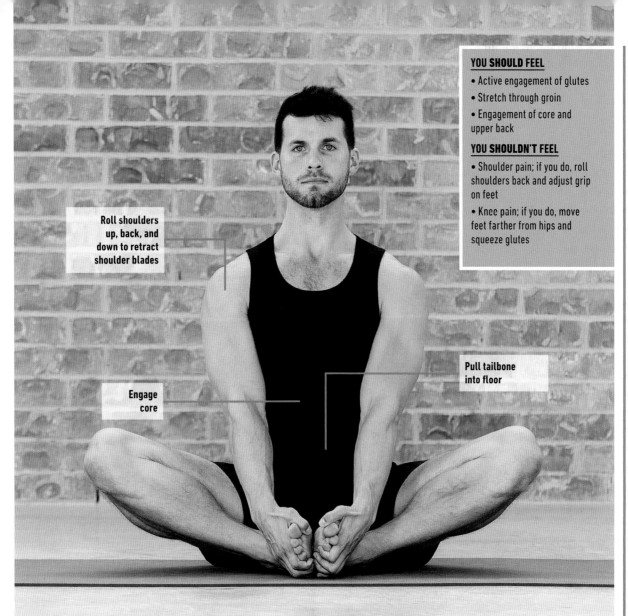

YOU SHOULD FEEL
- Active engagement of glutes
- Stretch through groin
- Engagement of core and upper back

YOU SHOULDN'T FEEL
- Shoulder pain; if you do, roll shoulders back and adjust grip on feet
- Knee pain; if you do, move feet farther from hips and squeeze glutes

Roll shoulders up, back, and down to retract shoulder blades

Pull tailbone into floor

Engage core

NOT THERE YET?

To help you sit more upright and reduce the required core strength, sit on a block, or place your hands just behind your hips.

2 Sit upright. Engage the glutes to squeeze knees closer toward the floor. Hold the posture, inhaling as you sit taller, and exhaling as you deepen the stretch in your groin.

SEATED TWIST

This seated stretch is a gentle way to strengthen the core and spine while improving glute flexibility. Seated twist maintains spine and hip health for people who do not find themselves in varied positions throughout the day. This is also useful as an active posture to relieve hip tightness from physical activity.

TARGET AREAS
• glutes • spine • core

BENEFITS
• Improves spinal mobility for reduced risk of injury and deeper twists • Strengthens core • Improves posture • Improves agility

1 Sit on the floor with both legs straight in front of you. Place your hands beside your hips, and use your core to lift your chest and flatten your back.

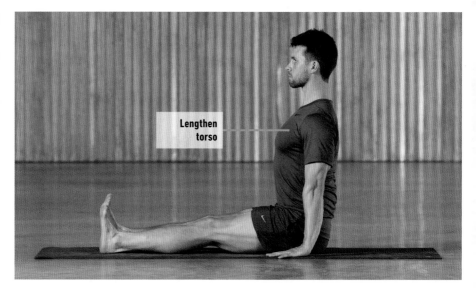

Lengthen torso

2 Cross your left leg over your right leg, and plant your left foot on the floor outside your right thigh, above the right knee. Hold your left knee with both hands, and sit up as tall as possible.

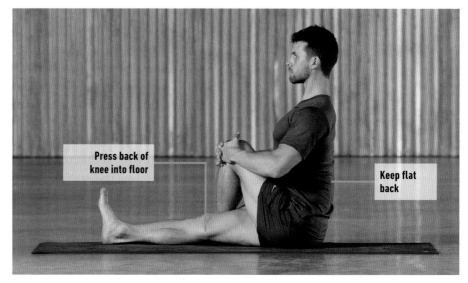

Press back of knee into floor

Keep flat back

YOU SHOULD FEEL

• Stretch in spine

• Engagement of inner thighs, hips, glutes, and core

YOU SHOULDN'T FEEL

• Pressing elbow into knee to deepen twist; if you are, use core for rotation

• Weight in arms; if so, ground yourself through hips and core

• Rounded or arched lower back; if so, engage core and don't twist as deeply

Press crown of head toward ceiling

Lift ribs away from hips and sit tall

Engage core

Keep heel on floor

PRO **TIP**

As you get stronger, focus on using core strength to maintain your posture and deepen the twist. Lift your hand away from your leg to test whether you are using your core.

3 Place your left hand on the floor and press the right elbow against the outside of your left knee to lift your chest and sit as upright as possible. Press down through your hips, engage core, and twist torso to the left. Hold the posture, inhaling as you lengthen the spine, and exhaling as you deepen the twist. Repeat on the other side.

CHILD'S POSE

This is an all-purpose pose to relax your body and release tension in your spine, back, and hips. It's a great cool down to return your breathing to normal, or a warm up to activate the core, upper back, and shoulders. Child's pose also helps relieve stiffness in the spine after sitting for an extended period of time.

TARGET AREAS
• hips • back • spine • shoulders

BENEFITS
• Relieves back pain and stiffness • Slows breathing and encourages post-workout recovery • Improves shoulder mobility • Straightens spine to improve posture

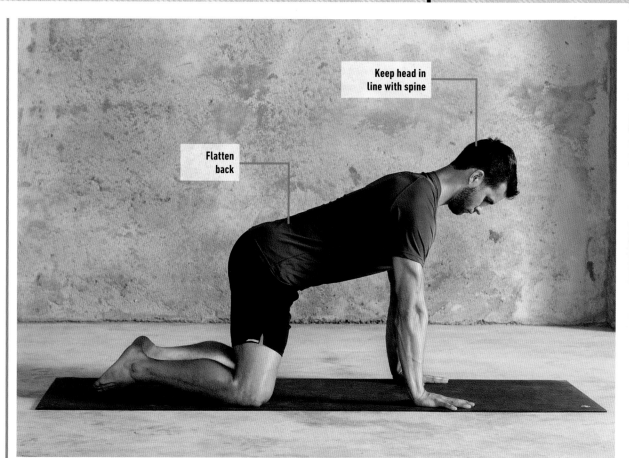

Keep head in line with spine

Flatten back

1 Start on all fours with shoulders over hands and hips over knees. Widen knees slightly wider than hip-width apart, and touch big toes together.

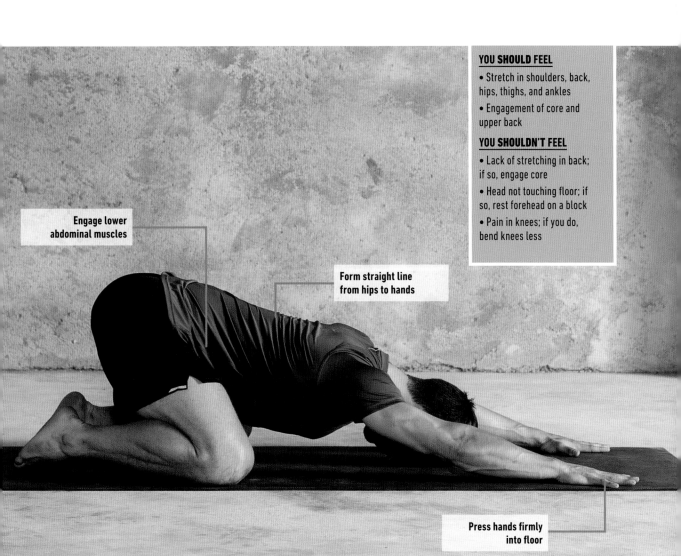

YOU SHOULD FEEL
- Stretch in shoulders, back, hips, thighs, and ankles
- Engagement of core and upper back

YOU SHOULDN'T FEEL
- Lack of stretching in back; if so, engage core
- Head not touching floor; if so, rest forehead on a block
- Pain in knees; if you do, bend knees less

Engage lower abdominal muscles

Form straight line from hips to hands

Press hands firmly into floor

PRO **TIP**

You can make Child's pose active or passive. To be more active, keep shoulders and arms engaged. To be more passive, relax elbows to the floor.

2 Shift your hips back toward heels as far as you comfortably can. Keep torso as long as possible. Keeping hips pushed back, walk your arms forward on the floor to stretch your back, and place hands shoulder-width apart. Lightly squeeze arms and shoulders toward one another, and firmly press hands into floor. Tighten lower abs, and draw ribs in. Hold the posture, inhaling to expand your chest and fill lungs, and exhaling to tighten abs and draw ribs in.

PLANK

The high plank position is one of the most basic yet effective postures for strengthening your core. Plank is great to warm up your body for exercise, build full-body strength, and strengthen your spine. It even helps increase testosterone levels, improve prostate health, and correct posture.

TARGET AREAS
• shoulders • arms • core • chest

BENEFITS
• Strengthens abdomen and upper body • Improves lower-back stability • Increases upper-body endurance • Strengthens prostate

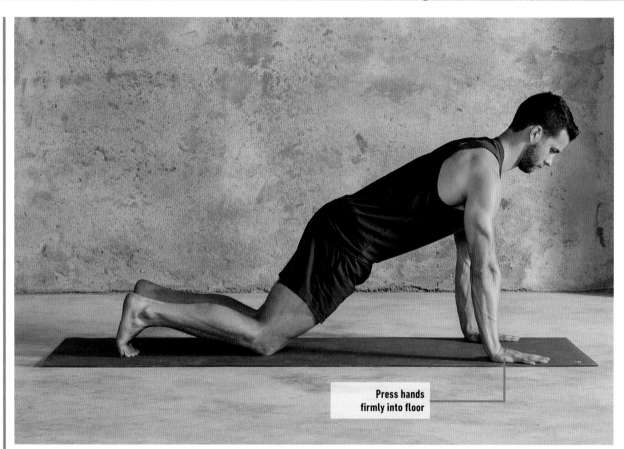

Press hands firmly into floor

1 Kneel on all fours with your shoulders over your wrists. Point your index fingers straight forward, and form an L-shape with thumbs. Push hands into the floor, and externally rotate arms so biceps face slightly forward and triceps wrap back. Tuck toes.

PRO **TIP**

As you press into the floor, externally rotate your arms for better shoulder engagement, as if you are opening a jar with your hands.

NOT THERE YET?

If it's difficult to maintain a straight line with your chest, keep your knees on the floor and practice engaging the correct muscles to build your strength.

YOU SHOULD FEEL
• Engagement of core, arms, shoulders, chest, and thighs

YOU SHOULDN'T FEEL
• Lower-back pain; if you do, make sure spine is straight, and engage your whole body
• Wrist pain; if you do, press down into area where fingers meet palms

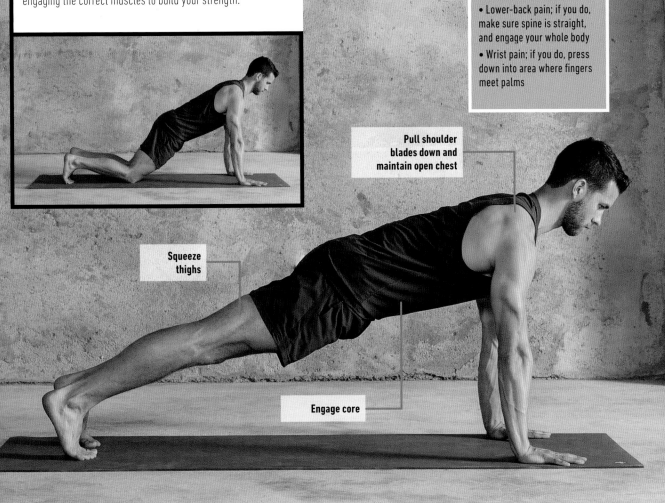

Pull shoulder blades down and maintain open chest

Squeeze thighs

Engage core

2 Lift your knees to form a straight line from your heels to your shoulders. Look slightly forward to properly align neck. Retract shoulder blades, and squeeze feet and hands toward your center. Hold the posture, inhaling to maintain the proper position, and exhaling to increase muscle engagement.

DOWNWARD-FACING DOG

This quintessential yoga posture stretches the calves and hamstrings, properly aligns the spine, improves shoulder mobility, and strengthens your hips, back, and core. It's great for athletes to improve lower-body strength and flexibility, and for weight lifters who need to stretch tight muscles and recover quickly.

TARGET AREAS
- hamstrings • hips • core
- shoulders • upper back • calves

BENEFITS
- Increases hamstring mobility
- Improves shoulder strength and mobility • Stretches calves to relieve ankle and knee tension

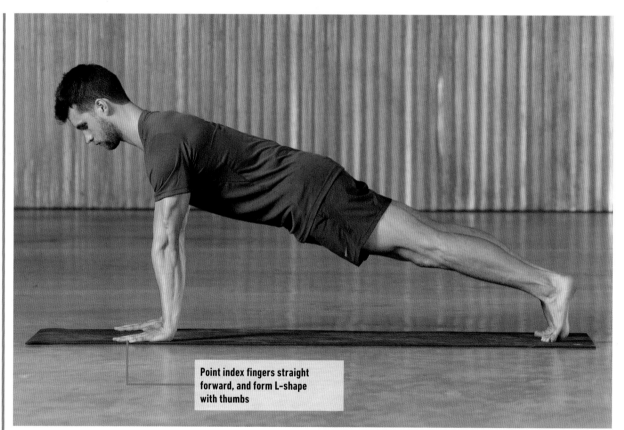

Point index fingers straight forward, and form L-shape with thumbs

1 Start in Plank (see p88) with your shoulders over your hands, core engaged, feet hip-width apart, and toes tucked. Lift hips to form a straight line from shoulders to heels.

PRO **TIP**
Once you're in the final pose, use a mirror to view yourself from the side, and focus on making your back flat. If you have trouble flattening it, walk your feet farther away from your hands, or bend your knees.

YOU SHOULD FEEL

• Stretch in hamstrings, mid- and upper back, and shoulders
• Engagement of quadriceps and core

YOU SHOULDN'T FEEL

• All your weight in shoulders and wrists; if so, pull shoulders away from ears and transfer weight to upper back, palms, and fingers

Squeeze core and upper thighs toward each other

Lengthen hamstrings to help flatten lower back

Slightly rotate thighs inward and squeeze legs toward each other

Squeeze arms and shoulders toward each other

Relax heels toward ground, lifting toes if possible

2 Lift your hips back and up to form a pyramid shape with your body. Focus on creating a straight line from hands to hips. Squeeze your upper thighs and abdominal muscles toward each other. Rotate biceps slightly forward to open your shoulders and release tension in the neck. Squeeze your arms and shoulders toward each other to engage the upper body. Relax your neck to look back at your feet. Release heels toward the floor to stretch the calves. Hold the posture, inhaling as you lengthen and lift, and exhaling as you deepen the stretch and increase engagement.

NOT THERE YET?

If it's difficult to engage the correct muscles, firmly plant your feet, hinge at the hips, and press your hands into a sturdy external support to form an L-shape with your body. Keep ribs drawn in, and avoid splaying open the chest. Notice what proper engagement feels like, then try on the floor.

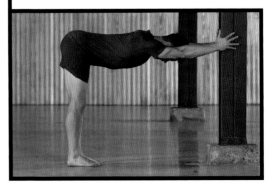

UPWARD-FACING DOG

It may look easy, but this posture is very advanced, requiring significant strength, mobility, and attention to the entire body. Upward-facing dog is a great warm up for any activity to activate the muscles of the core, spine, and hips, as well as a fantastic standalone exercise to build full-body strength and mobility.

TARGET AREAS
• core • back • shoulders • hips

BENEFITS
• Strengthens spine, back, core, shoulders, and hips • Improves spinal mobility and strength • Corrects posture

1 Start in Plank (see p88) with shoulders over your hands, core engaged, toes tucked, and feet hip-width apart. Lift hips to form a straight line from shoulders to heels.

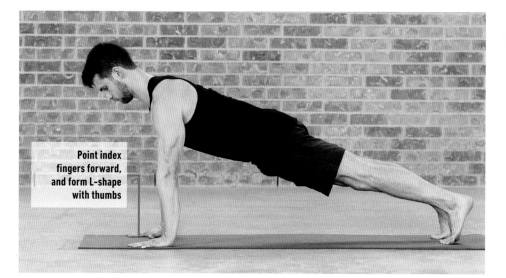

Point index fingers forward, and form L-shape with thumbs

2 Pull your body forward with your hands, and lower the shoulders to form a 90-degree angle with your elbows. Keep elbows directly over wrists, and keep the body rigid.

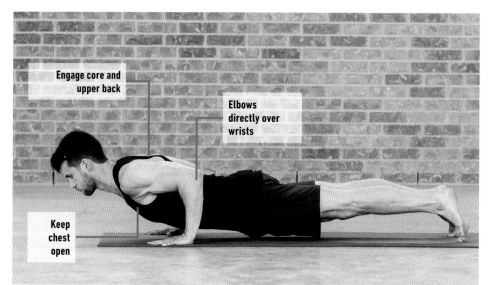

Engage core and upper back

Elbows directly over wrists

Keep chest open

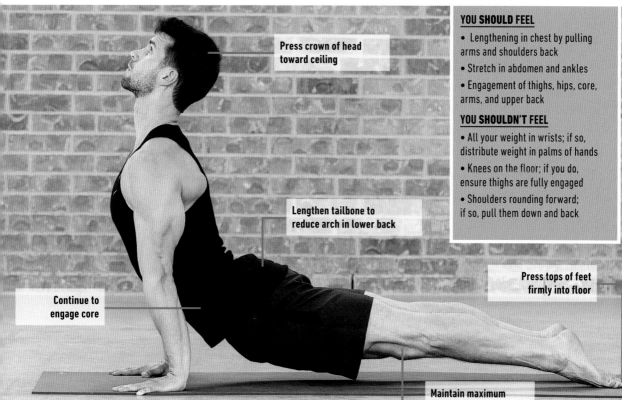

Press crown of head toward ceiling

YOU SHOULD FEEL
- Lengthening in chest by pulling arms and shoulders back
- Stretch in abdomen and ankles
- Engagement of thighs, hips, core, arms, and upper back

YOU SHOULDN'T FEEL
- All your weight in wrists; if so, distribute weight in palms of hands
- Knees on the floor; if you do, ensure thighs are fully engaged
- Shoulders rounding forward; if so, pull them down and back

Lengthen tailbone to reduce arch in lower back

Press tops of feet firmly into floor

Continue to engage core

Maintain maximum thigh engagement to lift knees

3 Inhale as you roll onto the tops of your feet, press tops of feet into the floor, and push your hands firmly into the floor to straighten arms. Open your chest and squeeze your shoulder blades toward each other. Rotate biceps forward so triceps wrap back, and squeeze elbows tightly to sides. Keep thighs engaged by squeezing ankles, knees, and inner thighs toward each other, and slightly rotate inner thighs so knees face straight down. Press the top of your head toward the ceiling, and slowly increase the arch in neck to look up. Hold the posture, inhaling as you lengthen the torso, and exhaling as you deepen the arch in your spine.

PRO **TIP**

Lower-body engagement makes this posture effective. Press down firmly into toes, tightly squeeze legs toward each other (from your feet all the way to your belly button), and maintain this tension the whole time.

NOT THERE YET?

If you have trouble comfortably combining all aspects of this pose, keep your hips on the floor. This builds the correct foundation for Upward-facing dog.

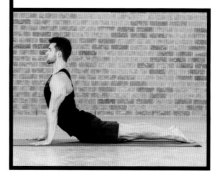

SIDE PLANK

Turn the plank position on its side to build upper-body and core strength, particularly in your obliques and shoulders, as well as the knees and hips. This posture also develops your balance. Use it as a warm up for any workout, or on its own to build strength and endurance.

TARGET AREAS
• shoulders • upper back • chest
• arms • core • hips • thighs

BENEFITS
• Improves core stability • Builds upper-body strength and endurance • Strengthens hips • Increases knee stability and strength

1 Start in Plank (see p88) with shoulders over your hands, core engaged, toes tucked, and feet hip-width apart. Lift hips to form a straight line from shoulders to heels.

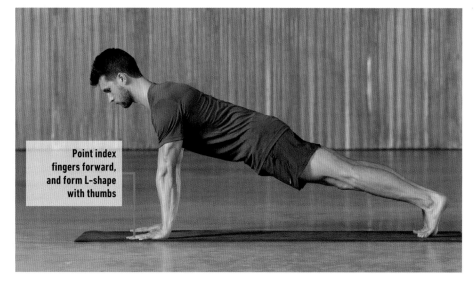

Point index fingers forward, and form L-shape with thumbs

2 Press down firmly into your right hand, roll onto the outside of the right foot, lift your left hand off the floor, and stack your left foot on your right foot. Flex your toes toward your shins. Place left hand on your left hip to stabilize hips and achieve balance, then lift hips as high as possible toward the ceiling.

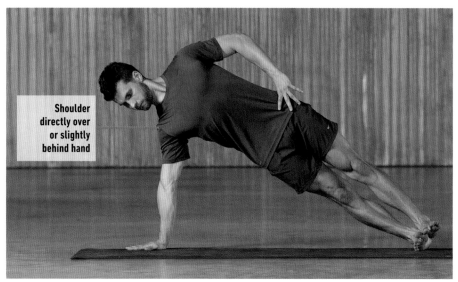

Shoulder directly over or slightly behind hand

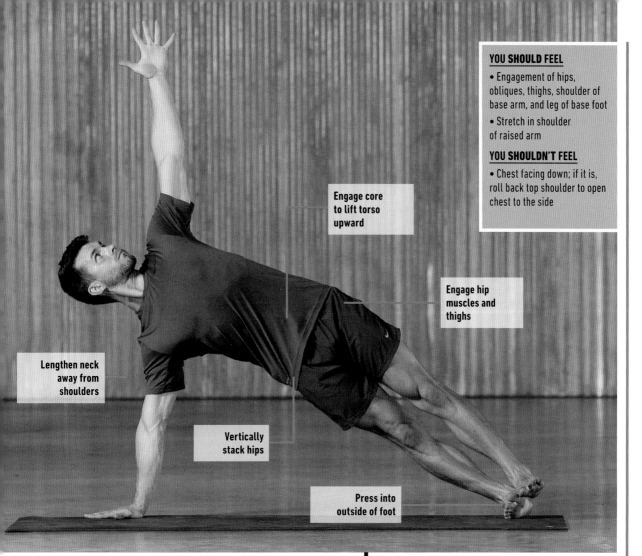

YOU SHOULD FEEL
• Engagement of hips, obliques, thighs, shoulder of base arm, and leg of base foot
• Stretch in shoulder of raised arm

YOU SHOULDN'T FEEL
• Chest facing down; if it is, roll back top shoulder to open chest to the side

Engage core to lift torso upward

Engage hip muscles and thighs

Lengthen neck away from shoulders

Vertically stack hips

Press into outside of foot

3 Extend your left arm toward the ceiling. Pull the crown of your head away from your chest, and rotate your head to look up at your hand. Reach your tailbone toward your feet so your back is straight. Hold the posture, inhaling as you lengthen your body, and exhaling as you reach your arm and hips higher. Repeat on the other side.

NOT THERE YET?
If it's difficult to support yourself, place your lower knee on the floor.

PRO **TIP**
Want more of a challenge? Lift your top leg toward the ceiling, keeping the foot flexed.

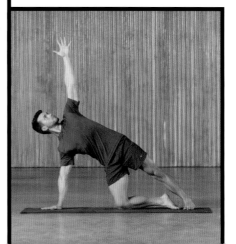

LOW PLANK

Low plank is a very difficult exercise, but it is also an incredibly effective way to build upper-body muscle mass and chest strength. This posture also helps prevent injury in the shoulders and upper back. As with any posture, it's important to focus on proper technique for the best possible results.

TARGET AREAS
• chest • shoulders • upper back
• arms • core

BENEFITS
• Builds upper-body muscle mass, strength, and endurance • Improves push-up form • Strengthens wrists and forearms

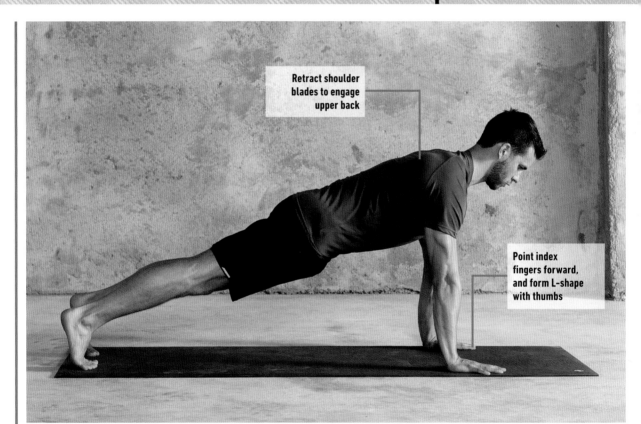

Retract shoulder blades to engage upper back

Point index fingers forward, and form L-shape with thumbs

1 Start in Plank (see p88) with shoulders over your hands, core engaged, toes tucked, and feet hip-width apart. Lift hips to form a straight line from shoulders to heels.

PRO **TIP**
Your shoulders should be neutral. Practice by doing Mountain pose (see p20), with your arms at your sides, palms facing forward. Notice the feeling of openness in the shoulders. This is how they should feel in Low plank, as well.

Keep shoulder blades retracted and chest open

Squeeze elbows into ribcage

Firmly engage core

Upper arms parallel to floor

NOT THERE YET?

If you don't yet have the strength to support yourself while maintaining proper form, lower your knees to the floor.

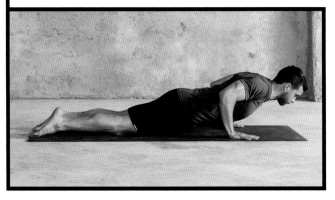

2 Pull your body forward with your hands, and lower your shoulders to form a 90-degree angle with your elbows. Lift shoulders away from the floor, and pull shoulder blades down. Squeeze elbows tightly into your sides. Gaze slightly forward. Hold the posture, inhaling as you maintain your position, and exhaling as you increase muscle engagement.

COBRA

This is one of the best spine and core strengthening postures in yoga. Cobra also improves lower-body and hip strength, builds muscle in your back, and helps prevent injury. It's an absolutely essential posture for people who sit often during the day, as well as for athletes to improve overall performance.

TARGET AREAS
• core • spine • hips • back

BENEFITS
• Strengthen hips, core, and spine
• Addresses root cause of lower-back pain • Improves posture

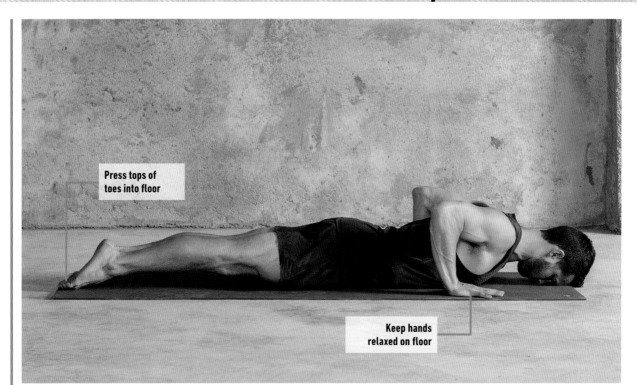

Press tops of toes into floor

Keep hands relaxed on floor

1 Lie on your stomach, and place your hands under your shoulders with your elbows pointing straight back, close to your sides. Spread your fingers wide and relax palms under your shoulders. Engage and rotate thighs inward so kneecaps point straight down and all toes are touching the floor. Squeeze your big toes, ankles, knees, and inner thighs toward each other.

PRO **TIP**

This is more of a hip and core exercise than a lower-back exercise. Focus on squeezing your legs toward one another as much as possible, and you'll have more success than if you concentrate on your back.

YOU **SHOULD** FEEL
- Intense engagement of entire legs
- Openness in chest

YOU **SHOULDN'T** FEEL
- Craning in neck; if you do, focus on lengthening neck and engaging core
- Glute engagement; if so, engage inner thighs, and turn inward
- Lower-back pain; if you do, lower back down, engage core and thighs, and try again with less arch

Lengthen entire spine

Engage mid- and upper back, and pull shoulders down and back

Continue to press toes into floor

Engage core

2 Press your pelvis and tops of feet into the floor. Inhale as you use your core (not arms) to lengthen spine forward and slightly lift your chest away from the floor. Press the crown of your head away from shoulders to look forward. Pull shoulder blades down and toward each other, squeeze elbows to sides, and use your hands to pull (not push) your body forward and up. Hold the posture, inhaling as you lift slightly higher, and exhaling as you increase engagement and maintain height.

NOT THERE YET?
If you feel back pain, focus on proper engagement of your core and hips, maintain length in the spine, and lift only a few inches instead.

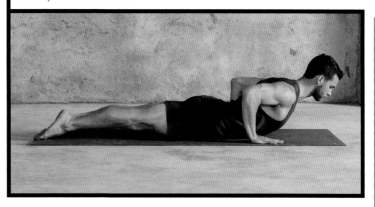

SPHINX

This is a great posture to strengthen the back while stretching the abs, making it the perfect exercise to counter a rounded spinal position, whether from sitting at a desk, deadlifting, or other fitness activities. Although Sphinx is an active pose, you can use it for restoration after a workout or sitting all day.

TARGET AREAS
• core • spine • mid- and upper back

BENEFITS
• Improves posture • Stretches abdominal muscles • Prevents lower-back pain from poor posture

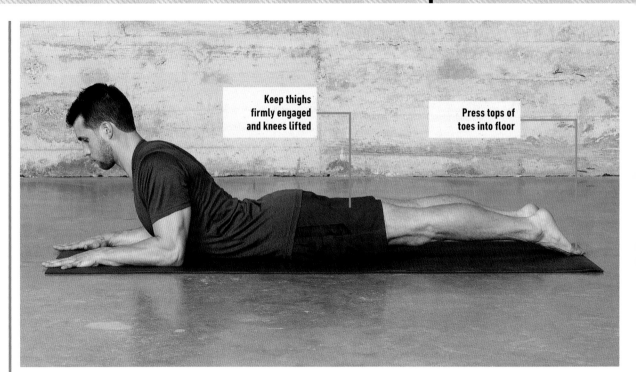

Keep thighs firmly engaged and knees lifted

Press tops of toes into floor

1 Lie on your stomach, and place your forearms flat on the floor, shoulder-width apart with palms facing down and elbows under your shoulders. Spread fingers wide, and press forearms, palms, and fingers firmly but lightly into the floor. One at a time, stretch your legs back as far as possible, pointing your toes. Engage your thighs, and rotate legs inward. Squeeze your big toes, ankles, knees, and hips toward each other. Press the tops of feet firmly into floor.

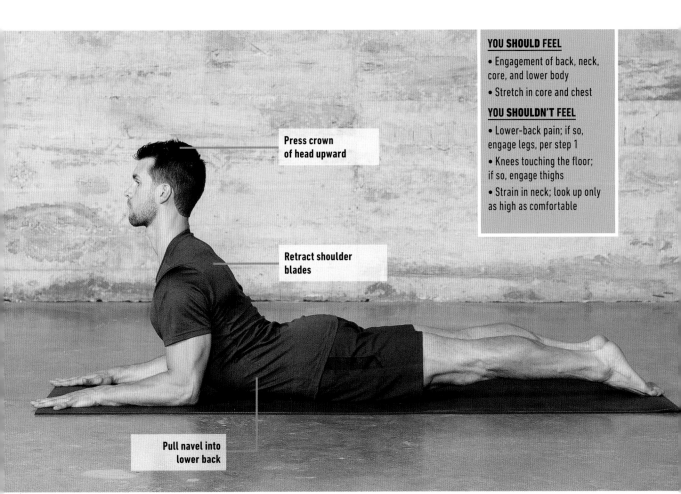

**Press crown
of head upward**

**Retract shoulder
blades**

**Pull navel into
lower back**

2 Use your forearms to pull your body forward and lengthen the torso, then press into your arms to lift your chest away from the floor. Engage your thighs and core to protect the spine. Press the crown of your head upward. Squeeze your shoulder blades toward each other. Hold the posture, inhaling as you lift slightly higher, and exhaling as you maintain height.

PRO **TIP**
This is a great posture to strengthen the mid- and upper-back, so focus on the muscle engagement to get the most out of this exercise.

DOLPHIN

This pose is extremely beneficial for improving shoulder mobility and building strength in the core and upper body, as well as stretching your calves and hamstrings. Dolphin helps maintain shoulder health for people with sedentary jobs, and is useful for athletes to improve upper-body performance.

TARGET AREAS
• shoulders • upper back • core • hamstrings

BENEFITS
• Builds shoulder and upper-back muscles • Increases shoulder mobility • Strengthens core • Improves posture

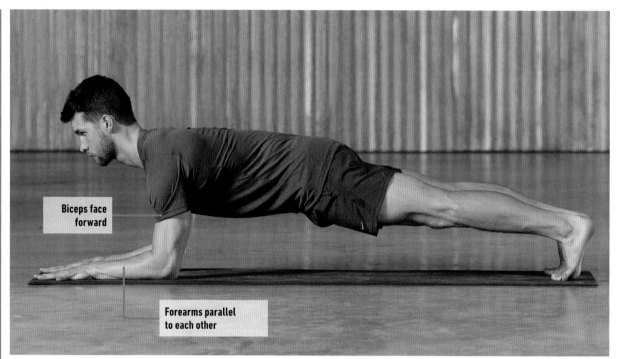

Biceps face forward

Forearms parallel to each other

1 Lie on your stomach, and place your forearms flat on the floor, shoulder-width apart, with palms facing down and elbows under your shoulders. Lift your hips and rise into a forearm plank with your toes tucked. Use your core to maintain a straight line from shoulders to hips.

PRO TIP
To develop active range of motion, as opposed to passive flexibility, focus on actively engaging your shoulders, core, and hips.

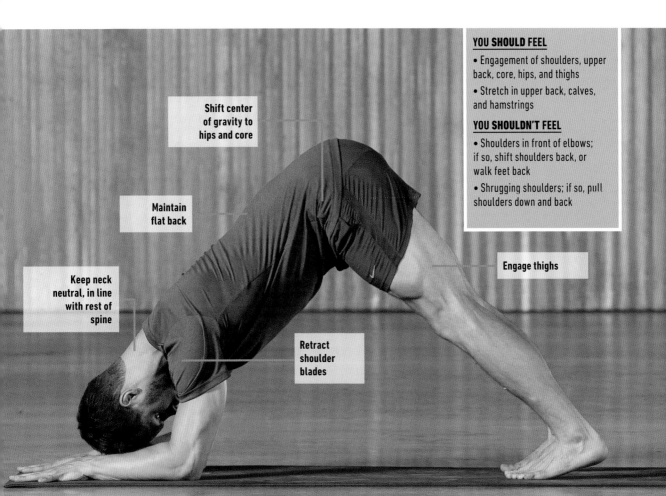

Shift center of gravity to hips and core

Maintain flat back

Keep neck neutral, in line with rest of spine

Retract shoulder blades

Engage thighs

YOU SHOULD FEEL
• Engagement of shoulders, upper back, core, hips, and thighs
• Stretch in upper back, calves, and hamstrings

YOU SHOULDN'T FEEL
• Shoulders in front of elbows; if so, shift shoulders back, or walk feet back
• Shrugging shoulders; if so, pull shoulders down and back

NOT THERE YET?

If your back is rounding significantly, place feet further away from your elbows. Bend your knees, and focus on flattening your back. Your legs will straighten more with time as your hamstring flexibility increases.

2 Walk your feet in toward your elbows, and lift your hips to form a pyramid shape. Reach your tailbone toward the ceiling, engage your quadriceps, and press your thighs up and away from shoulders to lengthen the spine. Relax your heels toward the floor. Squeeze elbows toward each other, keeping forearms parallel. Hold the posture, inhaling as you lengthen your spine, and exhaling as you deepen the hamstring stretch and increase shoulder and upper-back engagement.

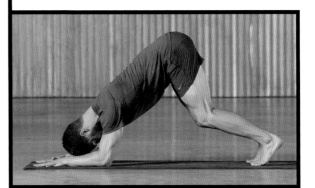

DOLPHIN

FULL LOCUST

This is a challenging, full-body pose that improves spinal mobility and strengthens your core, spine, and lower body. It's a great way for athletes and fitness enthusiasts to take core strength to the next level. Full locust should be a slow and controlled movement of every inch—don't jerk your body off the floor.

TARGET AREAS
• core • spine • back • hips

BENEFITS
• Strengthens entire back side of the body • Increases lower-body endurance and strength • Improves posture

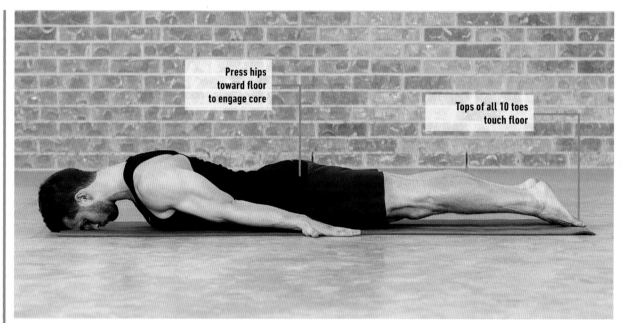

Press hips toward floor to engage core

Tops of all 10 toes touch floor

1 Lie on your stomach. Rest your arms at your sides, palms facing down, and straighten the legs. Relax your forehead on the floor. Engage your core and thighs, and rotate your thighs inward so kneecaps face down, and all 10 toes touch the floor.

PRO **TIP**
The key to this pose is focusing on length first, and then focusing on the lift. Press your toes and your head as far away from each other as possible, and then work on using your hips and core strength to lift. Depth comes with time and effort.

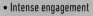

Press crown of head away from shoulders and gently lift chin

Maintain consistent arch through spine

YOU SHOULD FEEL

- Intense engagement of legs and core
- Engagement of back and triceps
- Stretch in chest
- Length in spine from tailbone to head

YOU SHOULDN'T FEEL

- Spine and neck pain; if you do, lower torso slightly and keep core engaged

Squeeze shoulder blades together

Keep knees locked

Point toes back as far as possible

2 Inhale as you lift your legs, arms, and chest away from the floor, and exhale to lengthen your body, pressing toes further back and head further up. Completely engage core and hips. Squeeze thighs to lock knees, and press toes back as far as you can, making legs as long as possible. Squeeze arms toward each other to engage the mid-back and open the chest. Hold the posture, inhaling to lift higher and increase arch, and exhaling to create more length from toes to head.

NOT THERE YET?

If you lack the strength to lift your entire body away from the floor, focus on developing proper muscle engagement first, and lift only slightly as you're able.

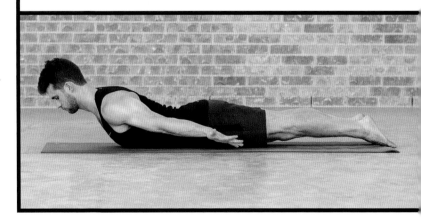

THREAD THE NEEDLE

This restorative posture stretches the rotator cuff muscles, relieves upper-back soreness, and releases shoulder tension. It's useful for athletes who use their arms often and for weight trainers the day after a back-focused session. It also relieves tension in the shoulders from day-to-day stress.

TARGET AREAS
• upper back • shoulders
• rotator cuff

BENEFITS
• Relieves upper-back tension that causes neck pain • Reduces risk of rotator cuff injury • Speeds upper back and shoulder recovery

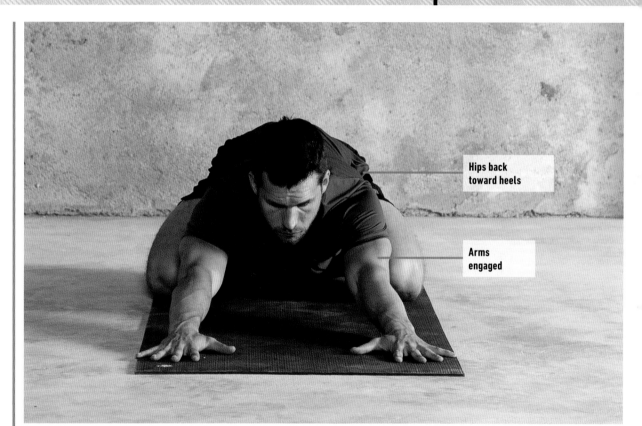

Hips back toward heels

Arms engaged

1 Start in Child's pose (see p86) with your knees wider than your shoulders, big toes touching, and hips shifted back toward your heels. Keep arms and torso long.

PRO TIP
This posture should stretch both shoulders at once. Make sure you press down firmly into the palm of your overhead arm to stretch that side.

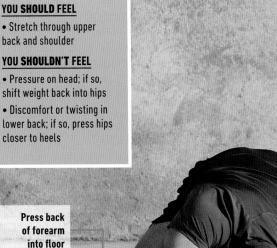

Neutral spine

Keep hips pushed back toward heels

Press back of forearm into floor

Pull crown of head away from shoulders

NOT THERE YET?

If this stretch is difficult, try it standing, instead. Bring one arm straight across the body, wrap the opposite forearm around the triceps, and lightly pull your arm to the side to stretch the upper back and shoulder.

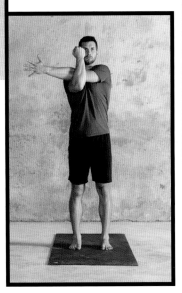

2 Slide your left arm under your right arm between the right hand and right knee, palm facing up. Press the back of your arm into the floor, and lightly pull it back to the left to stretch the left shoulder. Hold the posture, inhaling as you expand your chest, and exhaling as you deepen the shoulder stretch. Repeat on the other side.

THREAD THE NEEDLE

PIGEON

Pigeon stretches your glutes for faster muscle recovery, releases the lower back, and improves hip mobility. This stretch is one of the most important you can do for your back and your hips, leading to better jumps, sprints, and squats, and helping your back feel great throughout the day.

TARGET AREAS
• glutes • hips • lower back

BENEFITS
• Improves lower-body strength potential • Relieves lower-back pain • Prevents knee, hip, and spinal injury • Speeds up glute and hip recovery and muscle growth

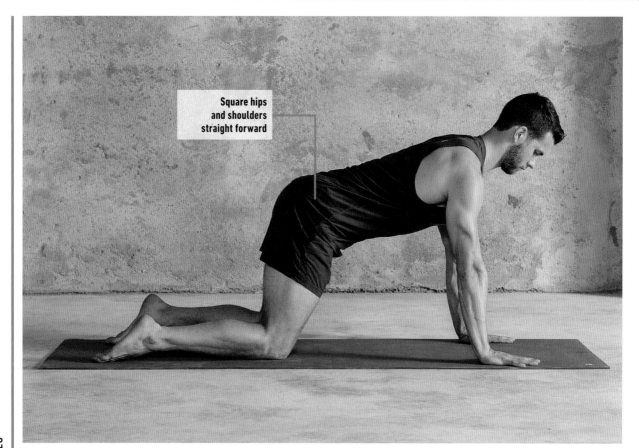

Square hips and shoulders straight forward

1 Start on all fours with shoulders over your wrists and knees under your hips. Untuck your feet.

PRO **TIP**

For an added mobility element, squeeze your knees toward each other and actively engage the glutes. To increase the intensity of the stretch, bring your front shin more parallel to the top of the mat.

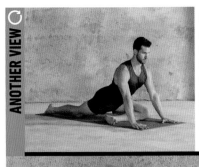

Notice how the inner thigh of the front leg faces up, and the outside of the shin touches the floor. This external hip rotation helps you increase hip flexibility by stretching the glutes more effectively.

YOU SHOULD FEEL

- Stretch in hip flexors, outer hip, and glutes
- Slight engagement of inner thighs and core
- Weight centered in hips; shift hips back, or use hands to help center your weight

YOU SHOULDN'T FEEL

- Pain in front knee; if so, flex knee to bring front foot closer to groin

Keep spine neutral

Keep hips square to floor

Right leg is straight back, not angled out to side

Rest on outside of leg, with inside of leg facing up

2 Slide your left knee up to your left hand, and bring the left foot across your body to rest between your right hand and right knee. Turn the left hip outward so the inner thigh faces up, and outer thigh faces down. Extend toes of right foot back as far as possible, releasing hips toward the floor as you do so. Rest hands a few inches in front of the bent leg, using your upper body to help square the hips straight forward. Hold the posture, inhaling as you lengthen the chest forward, and exhaling as you sink the hips closer to the floor. Repeat on the other side.

NOT THERE YET?

If the stretch is too intense or hips aren't level, place a block under front thigh, near the groin.

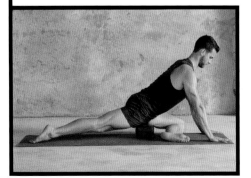

FROG

Frog is an intense restorative stretch for your groin and will greatly improve groin flexibility. Use it after an intense leg workout, at the end of a yoga session, or any time you're feeling sore. You'll want knee padding for this posture—use small towels or fold over the ends of your mat.

TARGET AREAS
• groin • inner thighs

BENEFITS
• Improves inner-thigh and groin flexibility • Reduces back pain • Promotes lower-body recovery • Prevents knee, hip, and spinal injury

1 Facing the long edge of your mat, get onto all fours and slowly move your knees outward, resting your weight on your hands and inner knees. Draw navel to lower back to flatten the spine.

PRO **TIP**
Continue to work deeper into the stretch for the duration of the pose. That may mean sinking a few millimeters deeper, or it could mean becoming more relaxed as you breathe without actually moving. The point is to keep progressing.

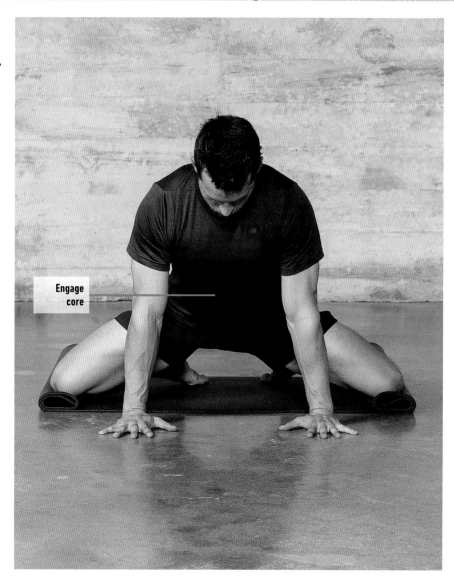

Engage core

YOU **SHOULD FEEL**

• Stretch in groin

YOU **SHOULDN'T FEEL**

• Pain in groin; if you do, decrease depth of stretch

• Pain in knees; if you do, use more padding beneath them

Keep back flat and core engaged

Look slightly forward so neck and spine are neutral

Keep ankles and shins parallel

NOT THERE YET?

If the stretch is too intense, stretch one side at a time, keeping one leg neutral. Start with your weight in the neutral leg, and slowly shift weight to the bent leg as your body adjusts to the stretch.

2 Shift your knees out as far as comfortable, then move shins and ankles directly behind the knees, so shins are parallel. Lower onto your forearms. Slowly shift the hips back until you feel a sufficient stretch in the groin. Hold the posture, inhaling as you hold your form, and exhaling as you relax deeper into the pose and shift hips further back.

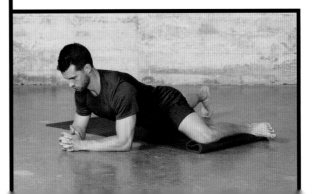

RECLINED TWIST

Twisting is an essential movement for maintaining a strong and mobile spine. This posture is one of the most basic twists you can do. Use at the end of a workout to speed up recovery, or the beginning of a workout to help open your spine for improved performance and reduced risk of injury.

TARGET AREAS
• back • spine

BENEFITS
• Relieves lower-back soreness
• Prevents spinal injury • Improves spinal range of motion • Promotes recovery of muscles surrounding the spine

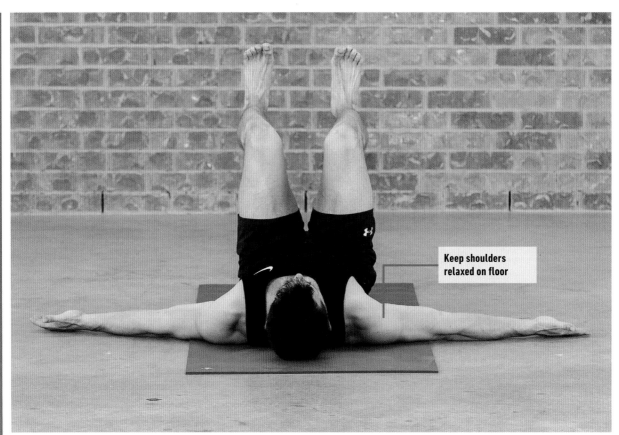

Keep shoulders relaxed on floor

1 Lie on your back. Lift your knees directly over your hips. Bend your knees and relax your legs. Extend arms directly out to the sides with palms facing the ceiling.

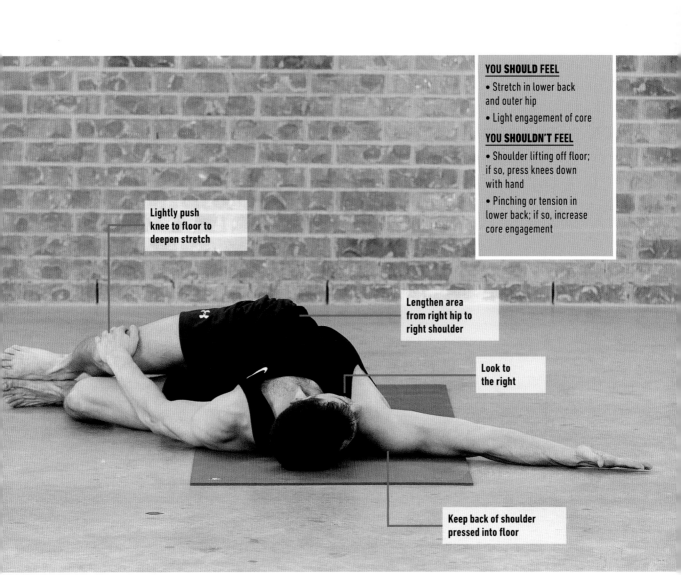

YOU SHOULD FEEL
- Stretch in lower back and outer hip
- Light engagement of core

YOU SHOULDN'T FEEL
- Shoulder lifting off floor; if so, press knees down with hand
- Pinching or tension in lower back; if so, increase core engagement

Lightly push knee to floor to deepen stretch

Lengthen area from right hip to right shoulder

Look to the right

Keep back of shoulder pressed into floor

2 Lower your legs to the left, keeping the legs stacked. Place left hand on the right knee. Use your core to twist, and pull your ribcage toward your core to deepen the stretch in your back. Press the crown of your head away from your shoulders, and turn to face the right. Hold the posture, inhaling as you maintain your position, and exhaling as you squeeze your core and deepen the twist. Repeat on the other side.

PRO **TIP**

If your spine is tight, it will take time for your body to adjust and your shoulder to comfortably rest on the floor, so don't worry too much if your shoulder doesn't rest on the ground.

RECLINED FIGURE 4

This is a great beginner's stretch to release glute soreness and counteract muscle imbalances caused by sitting. It can also alleviate pressure on the sciatic nerve by stretching the piriformis muscle, a small gluteal muscle. This stretch is a good alternative to Pigeon, because it requires less hip mobility.

TARGET AREAS
• glutes • hips

BENEFITS
• Relieves lower-back pain
• Eases symptoms of sciatica
• Improves hip flexibility
• Speeds up glute recovery

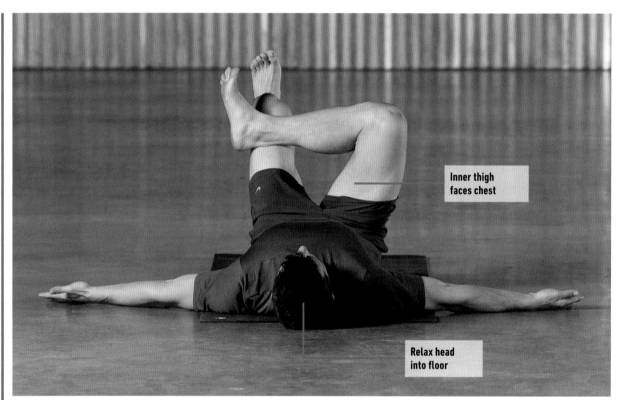

Inner thigh faces chest

Relax head into floor

1 Lie on your back. Lift your knees directly over your hips, and cross your right ankle over your left thigh to form a figure-4-shape with legs. Relax your arms. To protect the right knee, flex your right foot by reaching your toes toward your shin.

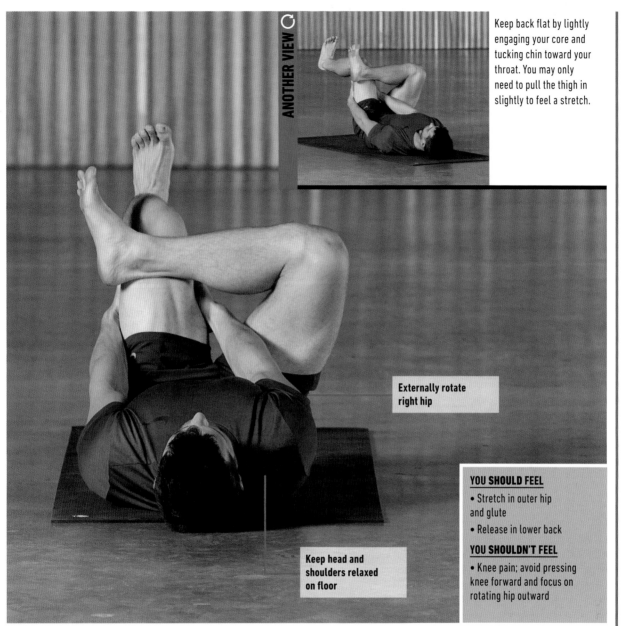

Keep back flat by lightly engaging your core and tucking chin toward your throat. You may only need to pull the thigh in slightly to feel a stretch.

Externally rotate right hip

Keep head and shoulders relaxed on floor

YOU SHOULD FEEL

• Stretch in outer hip and glute

• Release in lower back

YOU SHOULDN'T FEEL

• Knee pain; avoid pressing knee forward and focus on rotating hip outward

PRO **TIP**

Focus on the external rotation of your hip to stretch the glutes. Don't worry about pressing your knee forward.

2 Interlace your fingers behind your left thigh. Rotate your right hip outward so your inner thigh faces you. Gently pull the left thigh toward your chest. Squeeze the right glutes for a more active stretch. Keep your back, neck, and head relaxed on the floor by tucking your chin and pressing navel toward the floor. Hold the posture, inhaling as you maintain the position, and exhaling as you deepen the stretch. Repeat on the other side.

RECLINED FIGURE 4

BRIDGE

Bridge safely arches your back while strengthening your hips and core. This posture is essential for building stability in the spine and hips, especially for backbends. Do this exercise after a long day of sitting to balance your posture, or use this as a warm up to prepare the spine for a workout.

TARGET AREAS
• hips • core • spine

BENEFITS
• Strengthens spine, hips, core, and knees, and reduces risk of injury
• Warms up spine for safe exercise
• Restores balance to spine after prolonged sitting

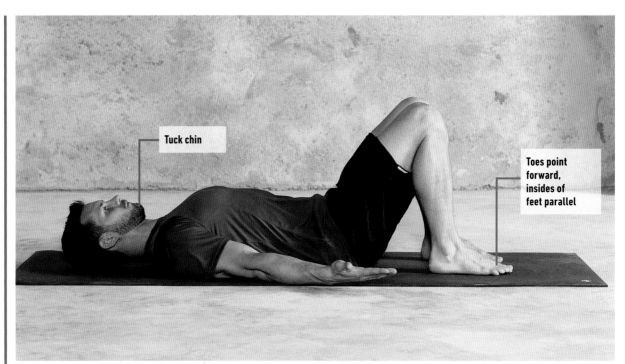

Tuck chin

Toes point forward, insides of feet parallel

1 Lie on your back and rest your arms at your sides, palms facing up. Bend your knees and plant your feet hip-width distance apart, no more than a few inches away from glutes. Tighten abs and engage core as you prepare to lift your hips.

PRO **TIP**
Focus on engaging the correct muscles rather than lifting your hips as high as possible. Think about squeezing your hips in toward each other to maximize glute engagement and strengthen hips as much as possible.

YOU SHOULD FEEL
• Stretch in fronts of hips and lower abdomen
• Engagement of hips, glutes, hamstrings, and inner thighs

YOU SHOULDN'T FEEL
• Lower-back pain; if so, engage core and glutes, and slightly lower hips
• Weight in neck; if you do, shift weight to shoulders

Keep knees hip-width apart, directly over ankles

Keep core engaged

Draw ribs in so chest doesn't splay open

Maintain neutral spine in lower back

NOT THERE YET?
If it's difficult to support your body with proper muscle engagement, lightly rest lower back on a block.

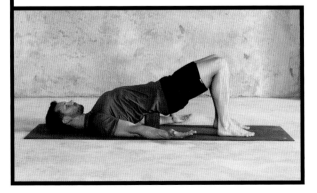

2 On an exhale, lift your hips slowly but firmly away from the floor. Squeeze the hips, glutes, and core to form a straight line from shoulders to knees. Reach your tailbone toward your knees to lengthen the spine. Hold the posture, inhaling as you lift your hips higher, and exhaling as you tighten your core.

HAMSTRING STRAP STRETCH

Using a strap allows you to passively stretch the hamstrings for a very effective release. This alleviates lower-back tension, speeds lower-body recovery, and helps prevent soft-tissue injuries of the hips and knees. It's a must for workout recovery, as well as for desk workers to ease chronic lower-back pain.

TARGET AREAS
• hamstrings • lower back • calves

BENEFITS
• Relieves pain and soreness in lower back and lower body • Prevents hamstring tears and pulls • Improves hamstring flexibility for deeper forward folds

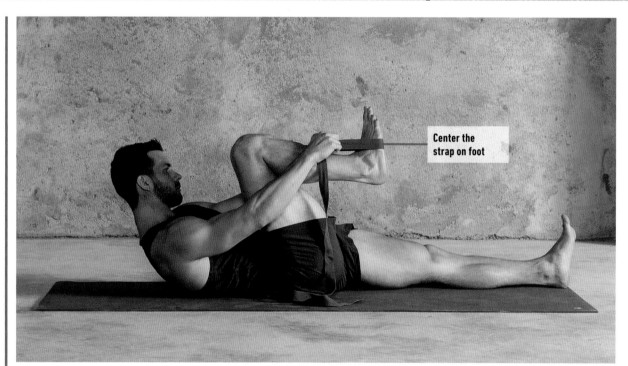

Center the strap on foot

1 Lie on your back. Position a strap on the arch of your right foot, and hold the ends of the strap with both hands. Rest your left leg on the floor.

PRO **TIP**
To get a better stretch in the hamstrings, squeeze the quadriceps of the lifted leg for the first 15 to 30 seconds of this stretch, and then relax the quadriceps to release.

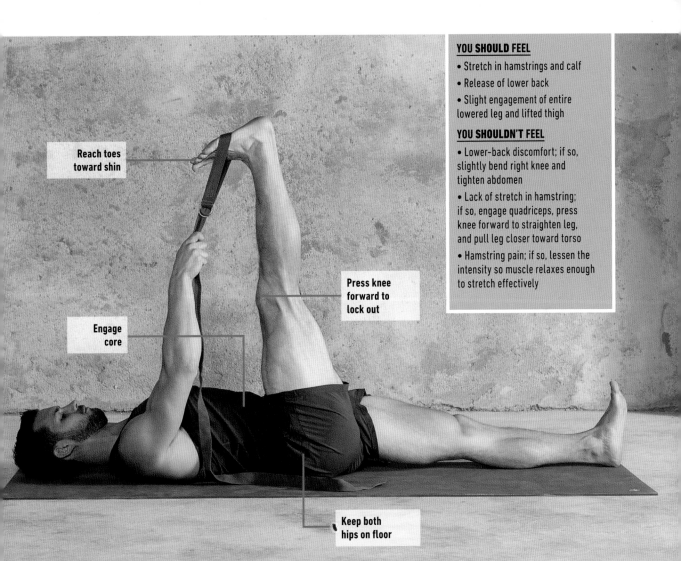

YOU SHOULD FEEL

- Stretch in hamstrings and calf
- Release of lower back
- Slight engagement of entire lowered leg and lifted thigh

YOU SHOULDN'T FEEL

- Lower-back discomfort; if so, slightly bend right knee and tighten abdomen
- Lack of stretch in hamstring; if so, engage quadriceps, press knee forward to straighten leg, and pull leg closer toward torso
- Hamstring pain; if so, lessen the intensity so muscle relaxes enough to stretch effectively

Reach toes toward shin

Press knee forward to lock out

Engage core

Keep both hips on floor

2 Keeping the left leg flat on the floor, straighten the right leg. Reach the toes of your right foot toward your shin and press the heel up to stretch your calf. Engage your inner thighs, and relax your shoulders, head, and back on the floor. Slightly tuck chin to keep neck and spine neutral. Hold the stretch, inhaling as you maintain the position, and exhaling as you deepen the stretch by pulling the leg closer to your chest. Repeat on the other side.

ANOTHER VIEW ↻

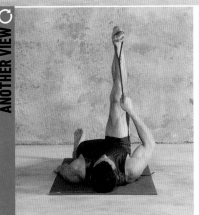

It's important to keep your hips and back neutral on the floor. You should bend your knee as needed to maintain proper form, or let your leg drop more toward the floor.

HAMSTRING STRAP STRETCH

INNER-THIGH STRAP STRETCH

Relieve tension in the inner thighs (adductors) and improve overall groin mobility with this stretch. This restorative exercise will reduce your risk of soft-tissue injuries in the hips, knees, and back. Use this after any workout to significantly reduce next-day stiffness, or after a day of sitting to release tight muscles.

TARGET AREAS
• groin • inner thighs • lower back

BENEFITS
• Releases lower-back pain caused by tight hips • Decreases risk of hip and knee injury • Promotes quicker lower-body recovery • Improves groin and inner-thigh flexibility

1 Lie on your back. Position a strap on the arch of your right foot, and hold the ends of the strap with both hands. Rest the left leg on the floor.

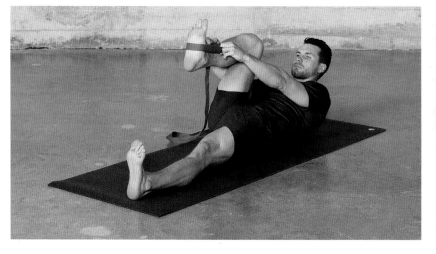

2 Straighten your right leg toward the ceiling until you feel a stretch in the back of the thigh. Reach the toes of your right foot toward your shin and press the heel up to stretch your calf.

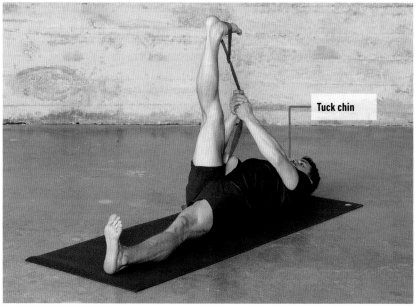

Tuck chin

NOT THERE YET?

If it's difficult to hold the strap, lie on your back with your legs parallel against a wall, soles of feet facing the ceiling, and glutes pressed into the wall. Slowly widen legs to intensify the stretch.

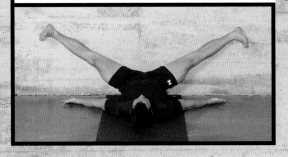

YOU **SHOULD FEEL**

• Stretch in inner thigh of lifted leg and outer quadriceps of planted leg

• Release of lower back

• Slight engagement of entire lowered leg and lifted thigh

YOU **SHOULDN'T FEEL**

• Hip of planted leg lifting off floor; if so, actively press that hip down

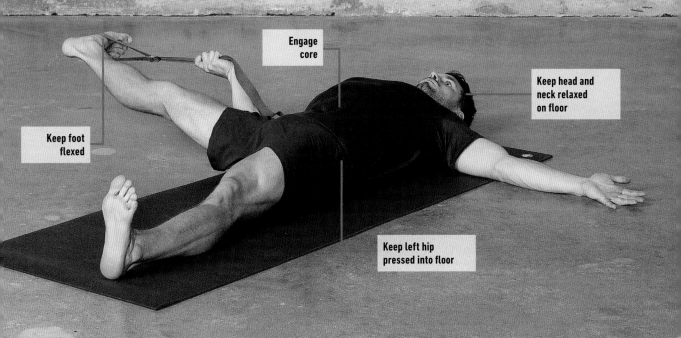

Engage core

Keep head and neck relaxed on floor

Keep foot flexed

Keep left hip pressed into floor

PRO **TIP**

For a deeper inner-thigh stretch that also builds mobility, squeeze the quadriceps of the lifted leg, and pull your foot closer to your shoulders.

3 Maintaining tension on the strap, slowly let your right leg fall to the right until you feel a stretch in the inner thigh. Keep left leg flat on the floor, actively pressing knee toward floor. Relax your shoulders, head, and back on the floor. Slightly tuck chin to keep neck and spine neutral. Hold the stretch, inhaling as you maintain the position, and exhaling to deepen the stretch by releasing right leg closer to the ground or pulling it closer toward your head. Repeat on the other side.

OUTER-THIGH STRAP STRETCH

This is a restorative stretch for releasing tension in the outer thighs (abductors), hamstrings, and lower back. This helps prevent injury in the knees and hips, and decreases recovery time after lower-body workouts. This is essential for anybody who works out often, as well as people who sit for long periods.

TARGET AREAS
- outer thighs • hamstrings
- lower back

BENEFITS
- Reduces risk of knee, hip, and spine injury • Relieves pressure in lower back and hips • Increases hip and thigh flexibility

1 Lie on your back. Position a strap on the arch of your right foot, and hold the ends of the strap with both hands. Rest the left leg on the floor.

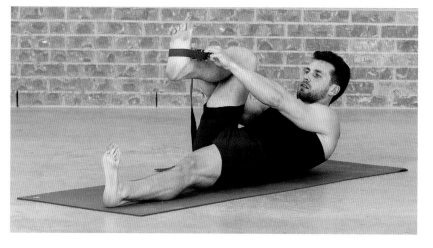

2 Straighten your right leg toward the ceiling until you feel a stretch in the back of the thigh. Flex right foot to feel a stretch in your calves.

PRO **TIP**
For the ultimate stretch in your outer thighs, focus on keeping the hip of the lifted leg planted, and your leg as straight as possible.

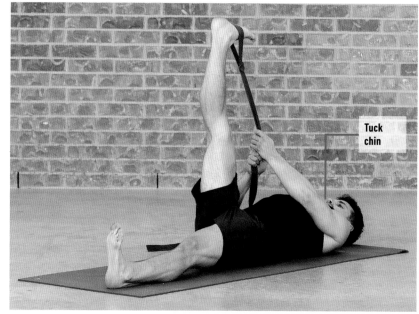

Tuck chin

YOU SHOULD FEEL

- Stretch in outer thigh and hip
- Release of lower back
- Slight engagement of entire lowered leg and lifted thigh

YOU SHOULDN'T FEEL

- Lack of stretch in hamstrings and outer thigh; if so, straighten lifted leg, and ensure hips are planted
- Twisting in lower back; if you do, make sure hips are planted evenly on floor

Keep foot flexed
Keep head and neck relaxed on floor
Keep hip on floor
Engage core

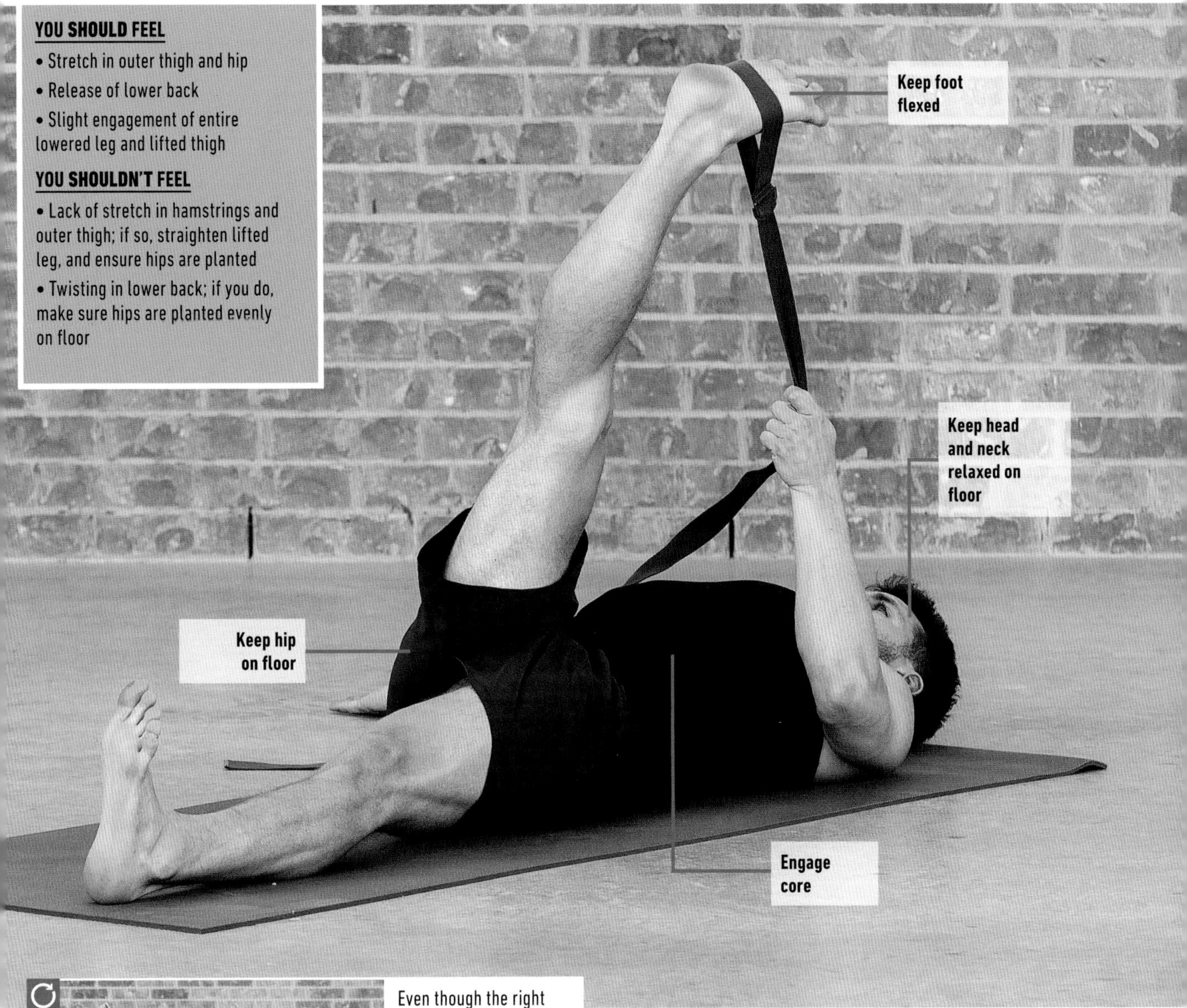

ANOTHER VIEW

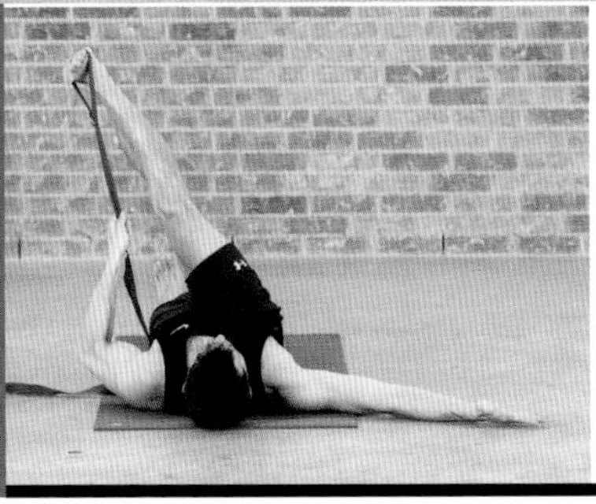

Even though the right leg falls across your body, be sure to keep both hips on the floor. You may not have to pull your leg very far to feel a deep stretch.

3 Slowly pull your right leg to the left across your body until you feel a stretch in the outer thigh. Keep left leg flat on the floor. Relax your shoulders, head, and back on the floor. Slightly tuck chin to keep neck and spine neutral. Hold the stretch, inhaling as you maintain the position, and exhaling to deepen the stretch by further straightening leg, or bringing it more across your body. Repeat on the other side.

HAPPY BABY

This is a great stretch for your groin to help relieve lower-back pain. Use Happy baby before a yoga workout to help warm up, or after a workout session to release muscle tension and speed up recovery. This posture is also perfect for when you want to move but don't feel like exercising.

TARGET AREAS
• groin • lower back • hamstrings • inner thighs

BENEFITS
• Releases lower-back tension and discomfort • Stretches groin and hamstrings • Increases hip flexibility

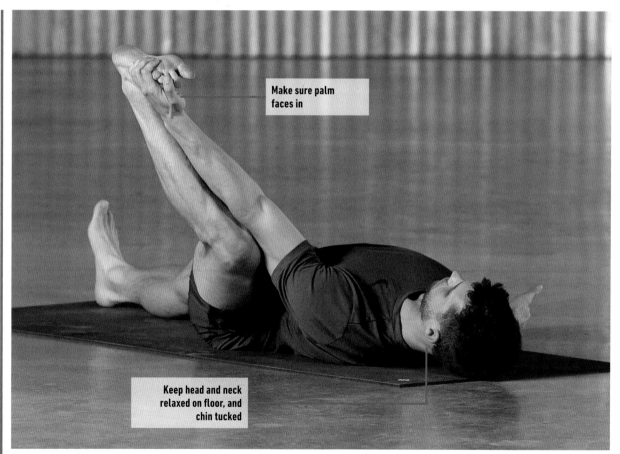

Make sure palm faces in

Keep head and neck relaxed on floor, and chin tucked

1 Lie on your back. Grab the outside of your left foot with your left hand, resting your elbow inside the knee.

PRO **TIP**
Roll lightly from side to side, and slightly bend and straighten your legs to achieve the desired stretch in your thighs.

YOU SHOULD FEEL
- Stretch in groin and hamstrings
- Release of lower back
- Slight engagement of quadriceps and upper back

YOU SHOULDN'T FEEL
- Lower-back pain; if so, bend knees more, and engage core

Keep lower back on floor

Retract shoulder blades

NOT THERE YET?
If it's difficult to hold your feet while retracting your shoulder blades, place a single strap across the soles of your feet, and hold the ends of the strap.

2 Grab the outside of your right foot with your right hand, resting your elbow inside the knee. Flex your feet by reaching your toes toward your shins. Press your feet up into your hands, and pull your feet toward the floor with your hands, creating opposing forces to deepen the stretch in your groin. Squeeze outer hips to drive knees outward. Relax your head, shoulders, and back, slightly tucking chin to keep neck and spine neutral. Hold the posture, inhaling to maintain the position, and exhaling to deepen the stretch.

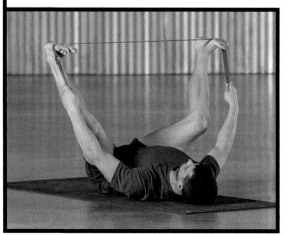

CORPSE

In any yoga class, this is usually the final resting pose, giving you a chance to release lingering tension and build your mind-body connection. Try not to worry about form; the important part is to relax your body and focus on your breath. Use Corpse to release everyday stress and boost your mood.

TARGET AREA
• total body

BENEFITS
• Releases tension in entire body
• Builds body awareness • Prepares body for quality sleep • Reduces stress • Lowers heart rate

1 Lie on your back, legs extended straight forward on the floor. Let your feet and knees turn out to the sides, releasing your hip muscles. Keep spine neutral. Relax arms at your sides with palms facing up.

2 Now it's time to release muscle tension. Shift your attention to your feet, and breathe deeply as you focus on the sensations in the toes; let toes relax a little more with every exhale. Continue in this fashion all the way up to your head, conducting a mental checklist of every body part, releasing tension as you exhale. After you've made it to your head, release any lingering tension by letting your body sink heavily into the floor. Close your eyes and breathe slowly, in and out through your nose. Inhale to expand your lungs and fill with air, and exhale to release more tension with each breath. Hold for a minimum of 2 minutes, or ten drawn-out breaths.

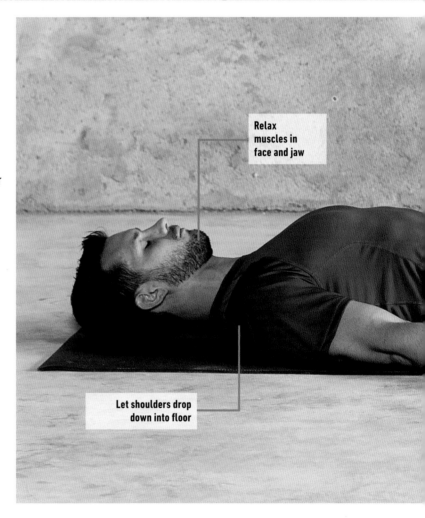

Relax muscles in face and jaw

Let shoulders drop down into floor

PRO **TIP**

You may be tempted to nap, but try to keep the mind active and your breathing slow and conscious. Mentally check in with each part of the body to build body awareness, and do your best to release all lingering tension. Strive for complete lack of muscle engagement.

YOU SHOULD FEEL
• No tension in your muscles

YOU SHOULDN'T FEEL
• Clenching of jaw
• Core engagement

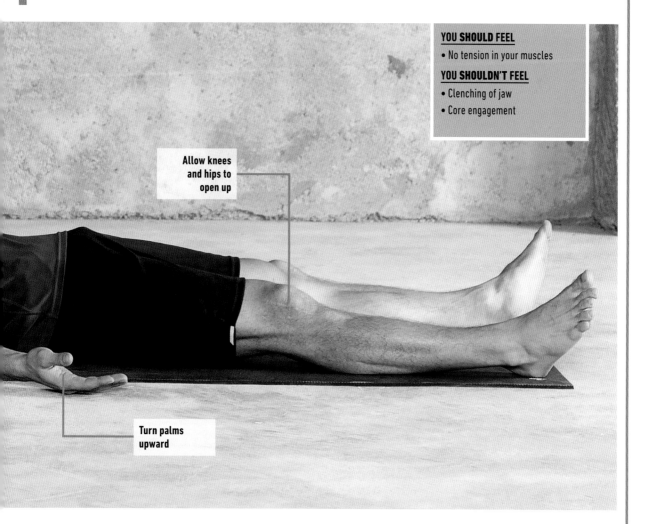

Allow knees and hips to open up

Turn palms upward

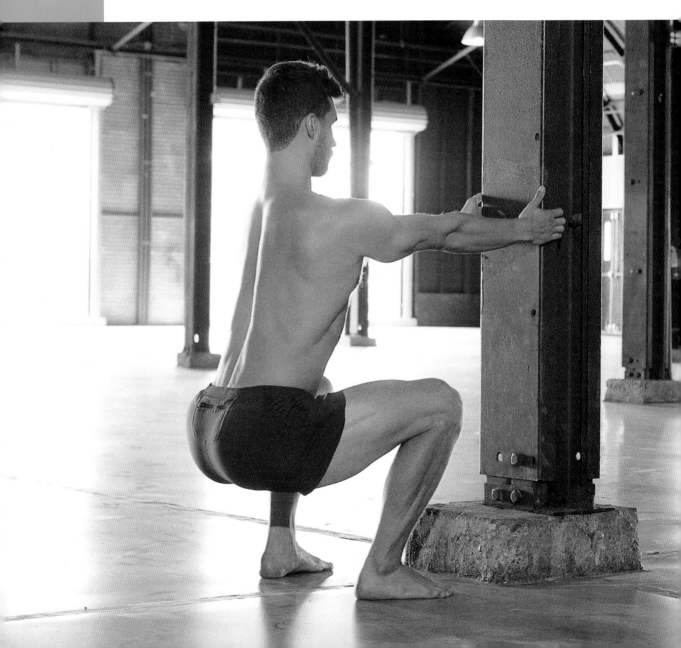

2 WORKOUTS

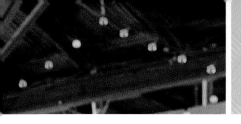

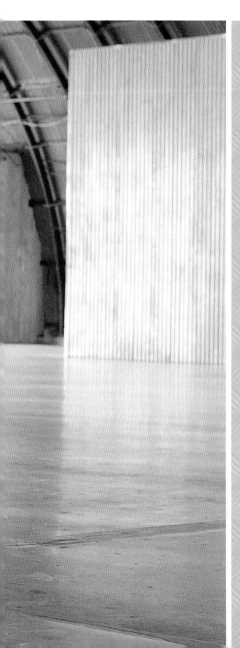

The following workouts make it easy for you to start exercising with yoga. They're organized into three categories, which will help you select the perfect routine.

Restorative workouts focus on relieving muscle tension. The less-intense postures improve your passive flexibility and relax your muscles. Breathe deeply, and relax into these poses as best you can.

Strengthening workouts use more strength-focused postures to improve mobility, balance, endurance, power, and muscle activation. Work hard, but maintain control over your body.

Restorative and strengthening workouts combine the two. They begin with postures that improve your strength and mobility, and end with a restorative section to speed recovery and help you get back to your workouts with less soreness, in less time.

Choose your workout difficulty level. The beginner and advanced levels on most workouts vary by the amount of time you hold the postures. Choose whichever track feels best for your body while still challenging you.

LAZY YOGA

This routine is for when you don't want to work out, but you still want to fit some movement in—no squats, lunges, or standing required. It's a great way to slowly wake up in the morning, as a substitute for a power nap later in the day, or as an evening routine to help you prepare for a restful night of sleep.

START

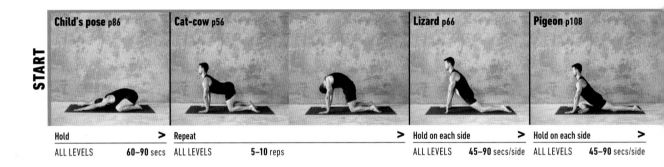

Child's pose p86	Cat-cow p56		Lizard p66	Pigeon p108
Hold >	Repeat >		Hold on each side >	Hold on each side >
ALL LEVELS 60–90 secs	ALL LEVELS 5–10 reps		ALL LEVELS 45–90 secs/side	ALL LEVELS 45–90 secs/side

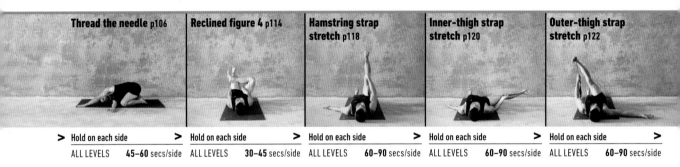

Thread the needle p106	Reclined figure 4 p114	Hamstring strap stretch p118	Inner-thigh strap stretch p120	Outer-thigh strap stretch p122
> Hold on each side >	Hold on each side >	Hold on each side >	Hold on each side >	Hold on each side >
ALL LEVELS 45–60 secs/side	ALL LEVELS 30–45 secs/side	ALL LEVELS 60–90 secs/side	ALL LEVELS 60–90 secs/side	ALL LEVELS 60–90 secs/side

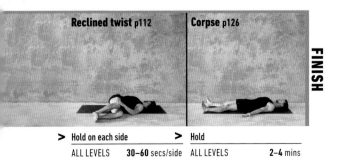

FINISH

Reclined twist p112	Corpse p126
> Hold on each side >	Hold
ALL LEVELS 30–60 secs/side	ALL LEVELS 2–4 mins

GOOD FOR

• Anytime you have low energy levels

• Relaxing your body for sleep

• Giving your body a quick charge
to restore energy

YOU WILL NEED

• a strap

GUIDELINES

• Hold the postures for the time given, or repeat for the reps
given, breathing consciously to work deeper into the poses.

• If the instructions say to hold on each side, do the left side
and then the right side in succession.

• Focus on deep, mindful breathing to relax into the poses
rather than pushing yourself too much. Try to make your
inhales and exhales last at least 4 seconds each, and build
up to 5, 6, 7, or even 8 seconds, if you can.

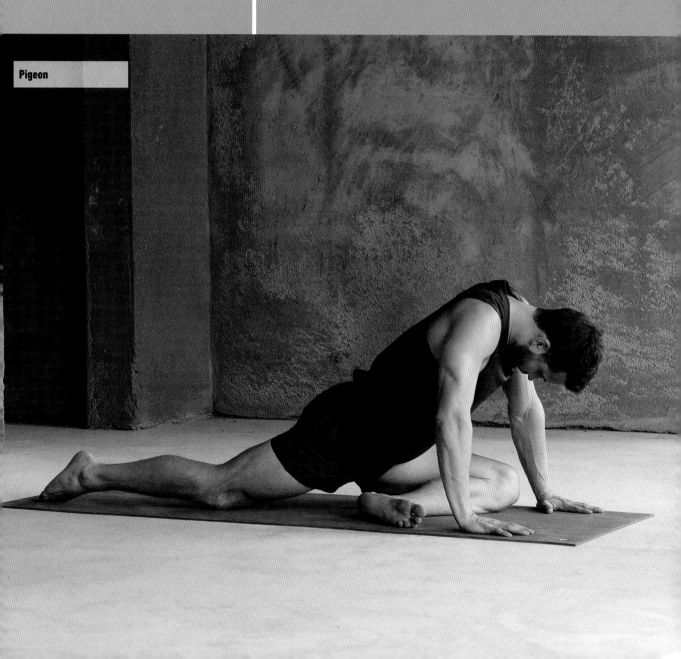

Pigeon

TOTAL-BODY SORENESS RELIEF

This is an all-purpose routine to relieve soreness, stiffness, and aching in your body. It's great for the day after a tough workout, relieving pain from sitting or inactivity, or easing weird kinks and aches in your body. You can also use this immediately after you finish a workout to help speed up recovery and reduce soreness the next day.

START

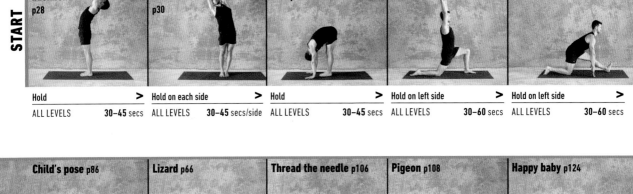

Standing backbend p28	>	Standing sidebend p30	>	Standing forward fold p21	>	Low lunge p58	>	Half split p64
Hold		Hold on each side		Hold		Hold on left side		Hold on left side
ALL LEVELS 30–45 secs		ALL LEVELS 30–45 secs/side		ALL LEVELS 30–45 secs		ALL LEVELS 30–60 secs		ALL LEVELS 30–60 secs

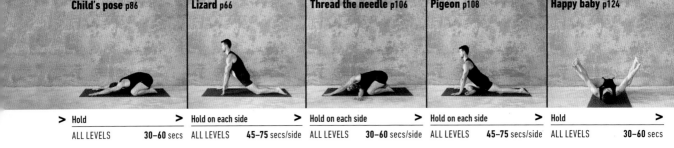

> Child's pose p86	>	Lizard p66	>	Thread the needle p106	>	Pigeon p108	>	Happy baby p124	>
Hold		Hold on each side		Hold on each side		Hold on each side		Hold	
ALL LEVELS 30–60 secs		ALL LEVELS 45–75 secs/side		ALL LEVELS 30–60 secs/side		ALL LEVELS 45–75 secs/side		ALL LEVELS 30–60 secs	

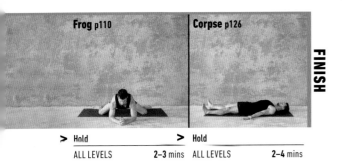

FINISH

> Frog p110	>	Corpse p126
Hold		Hold
ALL LEVELS 2–3 mins		ALL LEVELS 2–4 mins

GOOD FOR

• Athletes and fitness enthusiasts on the day after a workout

• People with chronic pain to gently relieve pain from muscle tightness

• Anytime you're feeling sore

• The day after a poor night of sleep

YOU WILL NEED

• a strap

GUIDELINES

• Hold the postures for the time given, breathing consciously to work deeper into the poses.

• If the instructions say to hold on each side, do the left side and then the right side in succession.

• If you're sore, you'll have to ease into these stretches. Start at a manageable level of flexibility, and slowly increase the depth of the stretch as your body adjusts and relaxes.

• Hold the posture as long as it takes your body to relax into it. If your body isn't relaxing, reduce the depth of the stretch.

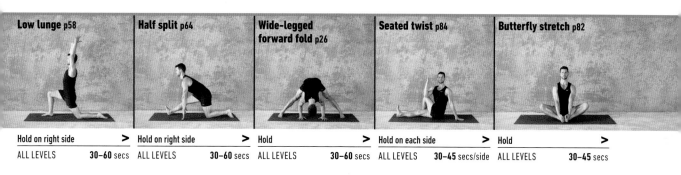

Low lunge p58
Hold on right side >
ALL LEVELS   **30–60** secs

Half split p64
Hold on right side >
ALL LEVELS   **30–60** secs

Wide-legged forward fold p26
Hold >
ALL LEVELS   **30–60** secs

Seated twist p84
Hold on each side >
ALL LEVELS   **30–45** secs/side

Butterfly stretch p82
Hold >
ALL LEVELS   **30–45** secs

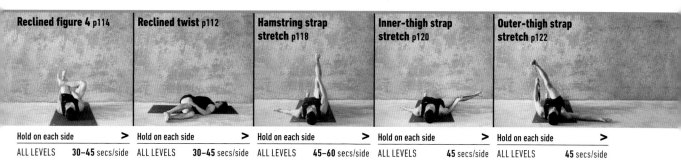

Reclined figure 4 p114
Hold on each side >
ALL LEVELS   **30–45** secs/side

Reclined twist p112
Hold on each side >
ALL LEVELS   **30–45** secs/side

Hamstring strap stretch p118
Hold on each side >
ALL LEVELS   **45–60** secs/side

Inner-thigh strap stretch p120
Hold on each side >
ALL LEVELS   **45** secs/side

Outer-thigh strap stretch p122
Hold on each side >
ALL LEVELS   **45** secs/side

BACK PAIN RELIEF

Use this sequence to immediately relieve spinal tension through a combination of strengthening and stretching. It stretches the muscles connected to your spine to directly relieve discomfort, and it removes pressure from the back by strengthening the core. As you hold the poses, keep in mind that back pain is usually caused by tight hips, spinal immobility, and a weak core.

START

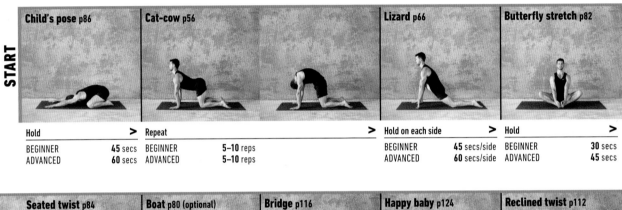

Child's pose p86

Hold >
| BEGINNER | 45 secs |
| ADVANCED | 60 secs |

Cat-cow p56

Repeat >
| BEGINNER | 5–10 reps |
| ADVANCED | 5–10 reps |

Lizard p66

Hold on each side >
| BEGINNER | 45 secs/side |
| ADVANCED | 60 secs/side |

Butterfly stretch p82

Hold >
| BEGINNER | 30 secs |
| ADVANCED | 45 secs |

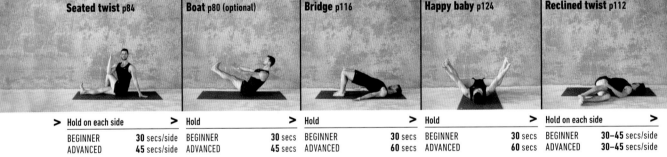

Seated twist p84

> Hold on each side >
| BEGINNER | 30 secs/side |
| ADVANCED | 45 secs/side |

Boat p80 (optional)

Hold >
| BEGINNER | 30 secs |
| ADVANCED | 45 secs |

Bridge p116

Hold >
| BEGINNER | 30 secs |
| ADVANCED | 60 secs |

Happy baby p124

Hold >
| BEGINNER | 30 secs |
| ADVANCED | 60 secs |

Reclined twist p112

Hold on each side >
| BEGINNER | 30–45 secs/side |
| ADVANCED | 30–45 secs/side |

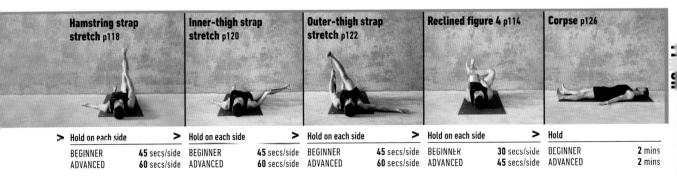

Hamstring strap stretch p118

> Hold on each side >
| BEGINNER | 45 secs/side |
| ADVANCED | 60 secs/side |

Inner-thigh strap stretch p120

Hold on each side >
| BEGINNER | 45 secs/side |
| ADVANCED | 60 secs/side |

Outer-thigh strap stretch p122

Hold on each side >
| BEGINNER | 45 secs/side |
| ADVANCED | 60 secs/side |

Reclined figure 4 p114

Hold on each side >
| BEGINNER | 30 secs/side |
| ADVANCED | 45 secs/side |

Corpse p126

Hold
| BEGINNER | 2 mins |
| ADVANCED | 2 mins |

GOOD FOR

• Athletes and fitness enthusiasts with exercise-induced lower-back pain

• Anyone with back discomfort

• People recovering from a spine injury

YOU WILL NEED

• a strap

GUIDELINES

• Hold the postures for the time given, or repeat for the reps given, breathing consciously to work deeper into the poses.

• If the instructions say to hold on each side, do the left side and then the right side in succession.

• Back pain is often caused by a weak core, so follow this sequence with a strength workout, such as Abs on fire (see p158), or Foundational core strength (see p156), to address the root issue and do more than just relieve pain.

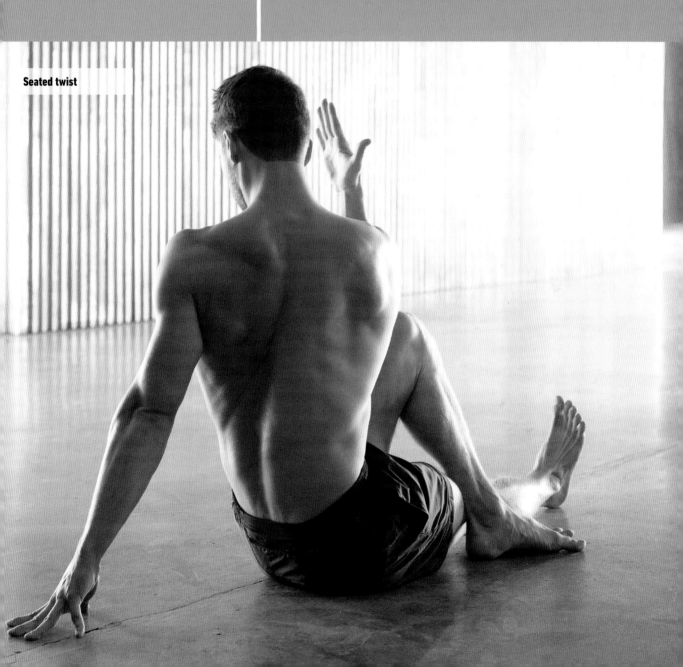

Seated twist

UPPER-BODY RECOVERY

This routine relieves soreness in your chest, shoulders, and back to immediately reduce upper-body discomfort caused by muscle tightness. The routine starts with a few postures to warm up your muscles, moves to lower-body postures featuring upper-body stretching, and then finishes with restorative upper-body stretches.

START

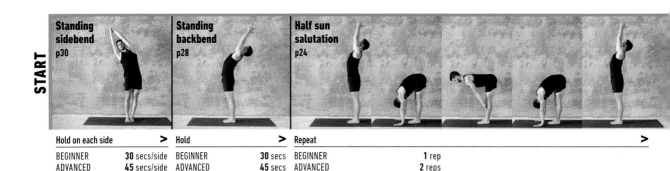

Standing sidebend p30		**Standing backbend** p28		**Half sun salutation** p24	
Hold on each side	>	Hold	>	Repeat	>
BEGINNER	30 secs/side	BEGINNER	30 secs	BEGINNER	1 rep
ADVANCED	45 secs/side	ADVANCED	45 secs	ADVANCED	2 reps

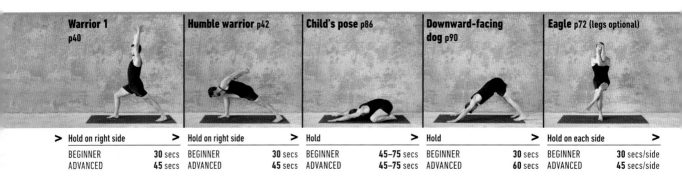

Warrior 1 p40		**Humble warrior** p42		**Child's pose** p86		**Downward-facing dog** p90		**Eagle** p72 (legs optional)	
Hold on right side	>	Hold on right side	>	Hold	>	Hold	>	Hold on each side	>
BEGINNER	30 secs	BEGINNER	30 secs	BEGINNER	45–75 secs	BEGINNER	30 secs	BEGINNER	30 secs/side
ADVANCED	45 secs	ADVANCED	45 secs	ADVANCED	45–75 secs	ADVANCED	60 secs	ADVANCED	45 secs/side

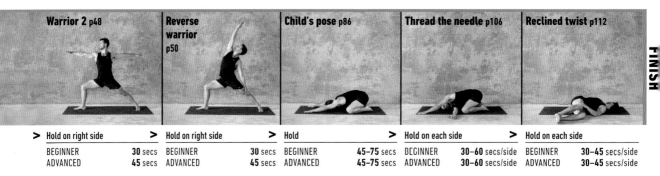

Warrior 2 p48		**Reverse warrior** p50		**Child's pose** p86		**Thread the needle** p106		**Reclined twist** p112	
Hold on right side	>	Hold on right side	>	Hold	>	Hold on each side	>	Hold on each side	
BEGINNER	30 secs	BEGINNER	30 secs	BEGINNER	45–75 secs	BEGINNER	30–60 secs/side	BEGINNER	30–45 secs/side
ADVANCED	45 secs	ADVANCED	45 secs	ADVANCED	45–75 secs	ADVANCED	30–60 secs/side	ADVANCED	30–45 secs/side

FINISH

GOOD FOR

• Athletes and fitness enthusiasts on the day after an upper-body workout

• Swimmers and other athletes who use their upper bodies often

• People recovering from upper-body injury

• People with high stress levels who hold tension in their neck and shoulders

GUIDELINES

• Hold the postures for the time given, or repeat for the reps given, breathing consciously to work deeper into the poses.

• If the instructions say to hold on each side, do the left side and then the right side in succession.

• Move as fluidly as possible from one posture to the next without resetting to a starting position unless necessary.

• Although these are full-body exercises, focus on your upper body during the postures.

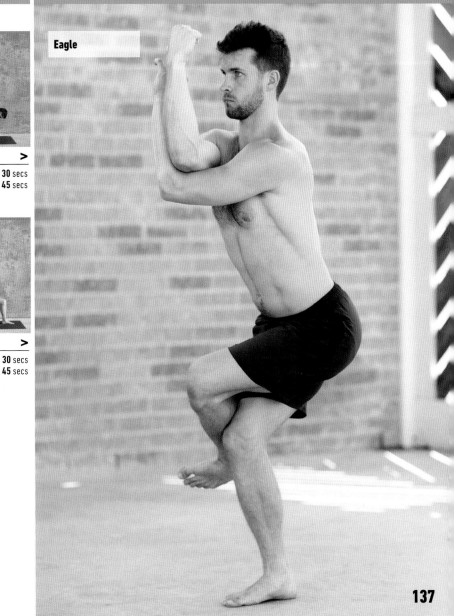

Eagle

Warrior 1 p40

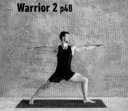

Hold on left side	>
BEGINNER	**30** secs
ADVANCED	**45** secs

Humble warrior p42

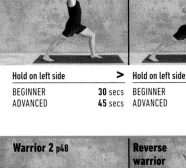

Hold on left side	>
BEGINNER	**30** secs
ADVANCED	**45** secs

Warrior 2 p48

Hold on left side	>
BEGINNER	**30** secs
ADVANCED	**45** secs

Reverse warrior p50

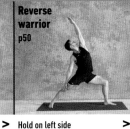

Hold on left side	>
BEGINNER	**30** secs
ADVANCED	**45** secs

LEG-DAY RECOVERY

This routine starts with a few postures to get your muscles warm, then moves to restorative stretches to relieve tension and soreness in your lower body. Do this routine to promote recovery from an intense workout or to help prevent injuries caused by over-training.

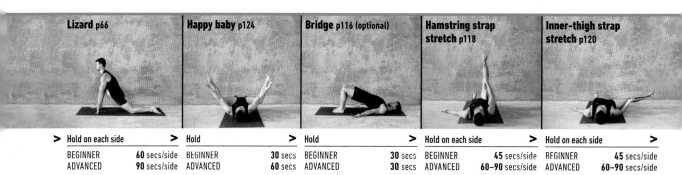

START

Bridge p116	Seated twist p84	Butterfly stretch p82	Cat-cow p56 (optional)
Hold >	**Hold on each side** >	**Hold** >	**Repeat** >
BEGINNER 30 secs	BEGINNER 30 secs/side	BEGINNER 30 secs	BEGINNER 5–10 reps
ADVANCED 45 secs	ADVANCED 45 secs/side	ADVANCED 60 secs	ADVANCED 5–10 reps

Half sun salutation p24 (continued)				Warrior 1 p40	Pyramid p44
>			>	**Hold on left side** >	**Hold on left side** >
				BEGINNER 30 secs	BEGINNER 30 secs
				ADVANCED 45 secs	ADVANCED 45 secs

Lizard p66	Happy baby p124	Bridge p116 (optional)	Hamstring strap stretch p118	Inner-thigh strap stretch p120
> **Hold on each side** >	**Hold** >	**Hold** >	**Hold on each side** >	**Hold on each side** >
BEGINNER 60 secs/side	BEGINNER 30 secs	BEGINNER 30 secs	BEGINNER 45 secs/side	BEGINNER 45 secs/side
ADVANCED 90 secs/side	ADVANCED 60 secs	ADVANCED 30 secs	ADVANCED 60–90 secs/side	ADVANCED 60–90 secs/side

GOOD FOR

- People with back pain due to tight hips
- Athletes, fitness enthusiasts, runners, cyclists, and endurance athletes on the day after a lower-body workout
- People with injury, pain, or tenderness in ankles, knees, or hips

YOU WILL NEED

- a strap • a block to modify if you're new to yoga or less flexible

GUIDELINES

- Hold the postures for the time given, or repeat for the reps given, breathing consciously to work deeper into the poses.
- If the instructions say to hold on each side, do the left side and then the right side in succession.
- Move as fluidly as possible from one posture to the next without resetting to a starting position unless necessary.
- This is a recovery workout, so focus on deep breathing to release muscle tension and promote quick recovery.

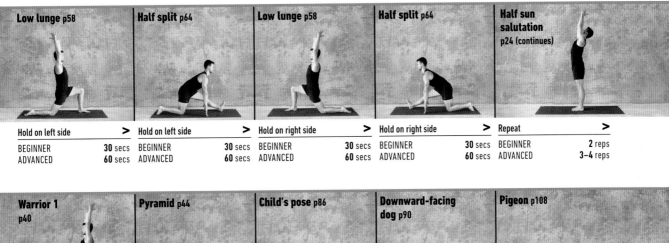

Low lunge p58

Hold on left side	>
BEGINNER	30 secs
ADVANCED	60 secs

Half split p64

Hold on left side	>
BEGINNER	30 secs
ADVANCED	60 secs

Low lunge p58

Hold on right side	>
BEGINNER	30 secs
ADVANCED	60 secs

Half split p64

Hold on right side	>
BEGINNER	30 secs
ADVANCED	60 secs

Half sun salutation p24 (continues)

Repeat	>
BEGINNER	2 reps
ADVANCED	3–4 reps

Warrior 1 p40

Hold on right side	>
BEGINNER	30 secs
ADVANCED	45 secs

Pyramid p44

Hold on right side	>
BEGINNER	30 secs
ADVANCED	45 secs

Child's pose p86

Hold	>
BEGINNER	30–60 secs
ADVANCED	30–60 secs

Downward-facing dog p90

Hold	>
BEGINNER	30 secs
ADVANCED	60 secs

Pigeon p108

Hold on each side	>
BEGINNER	60 secs/side
ADVANCED	90 secs/side

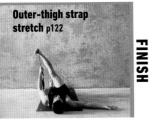

FINISH

Outer-thigh strap stretch p122

Hold on each side	
BEGINNER	45 secs/side
ADVANCED	60–90 secs/side

KNEE AND ANKLE
PAIN RELIEF

Stretch the muscles that connect to your ankles and knees to improve lower-body flexibility, relieve pain in your joints, and jump-start recovery. Although this is a restorative routine, be sure to engage the correct muscles to help you stretch safely and maintain proper form.

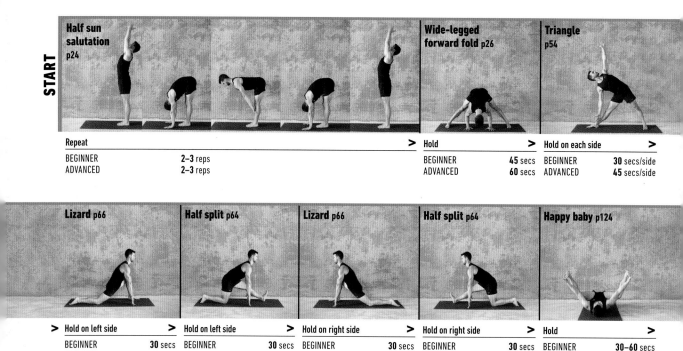

START

Half sun salutation p24

Wide-legged forward fold p26

Triangle p54

Repeat	>	Hold	>	Hold on each side	>
BEGINNER	2–3 reps	BEGINNER	45 secs	BEGINNER	30 secs/side
ADVANCED	2–3 reps	ADVANCED	60 secs	ADVANCED	45 secs/side

Lizard p66

Half split p64

Lizard p66

Half split p64

Happy baby p124

> Hold on left side	>	Hold on left side	>	Hold on right side	>	Hold on right side	>	Hold	>
BEGINNER	30 secs	BEGINNER	30 secs	BEGINNER	30 secs	BEGINNER	30 secs	BEGINNER	30–60 secs
ADVANCED	45 secs	ADVANCED	45 secs	ADVANCED	45 secs	ADVANCED	45 secs	ADVANCED	30–60 secs

Bridge p116

Hamstring strap stretch p118

Inner-thigh strap stretch p120

Outer-thigh strap stretch p122

FINISH

> Hold	>	Hold on each side	>	Hold on each side	>	Hold on each side	
BEGINNER	30 secs	BEGINNER	45 secs/side	BEGINNER	45 secs/side	BEGINNER	45 secs/side
ADVANCED	45 secs	ADVANCED	60 secs/side	ADVANCED	60 secs/side	ADVANCED	60 secs/side

GOOD FOR

• The day after a high-impact lower-body workout, such as running, calisthenics, HIIT, or weight training

• Relieving tightness or stiffness in the lower body

• Recovering more quickly for an important fitness event or competition

YOU WILL NEED

• a strap

GUIDELINES

• Hold the postures for the time given, or repeat for the reps given, breathing consciously to work deeper into the poses.

• If the instructions say to hold on each side, do the left side and then the right side in succession.

• Move as fluidly as possible from one posture to the next without resetting to a starting position unless necessary.

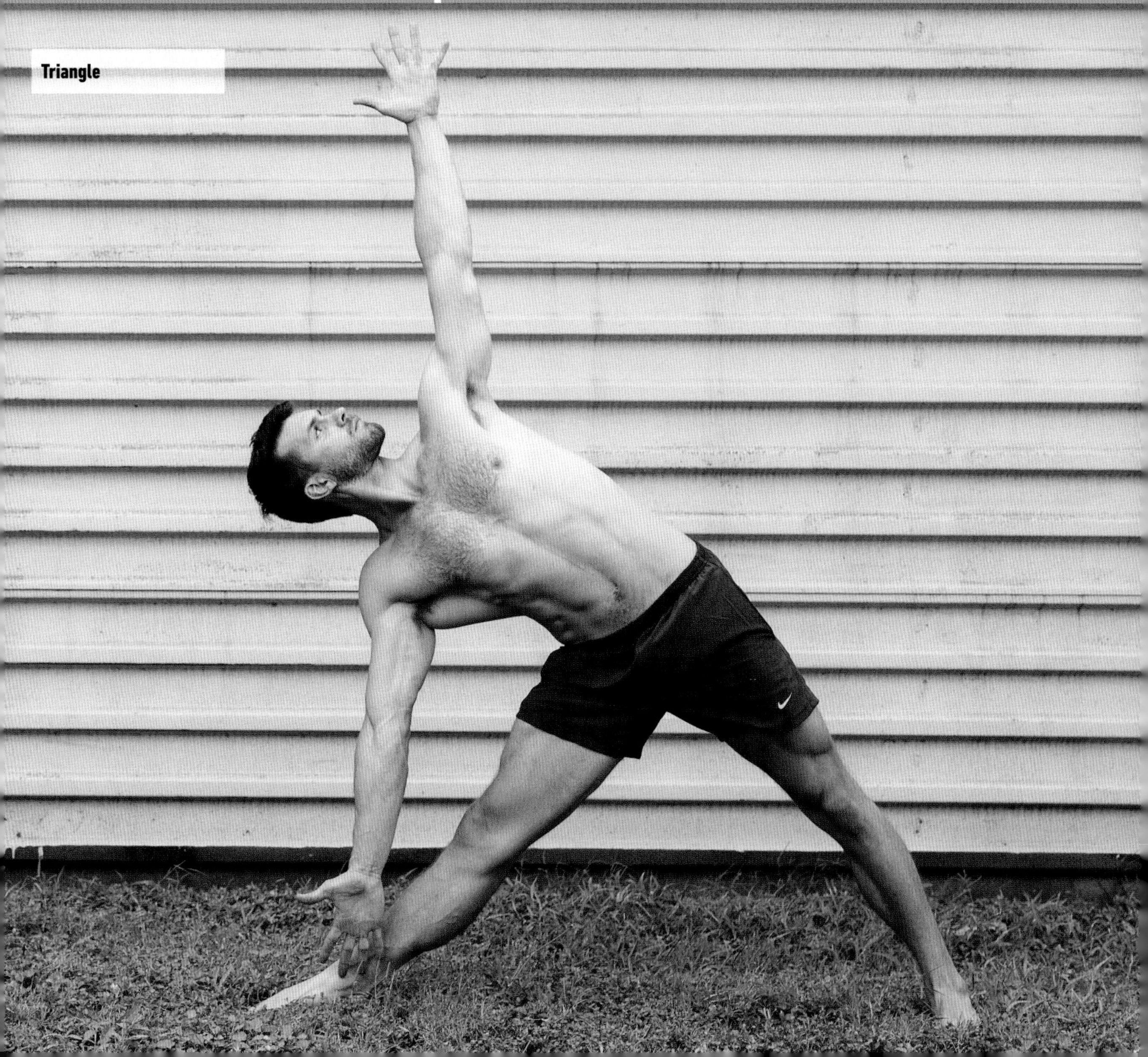

Triangle

STANDING RELIEF

This routine is good for days when you've been active and on your feet for a long time. These postures place your body in positions you won't typically find yourself when standing, which helps to correct muscle imbalances, improve spinal alignment, stretch tight and overworked muscles, and even build strength.

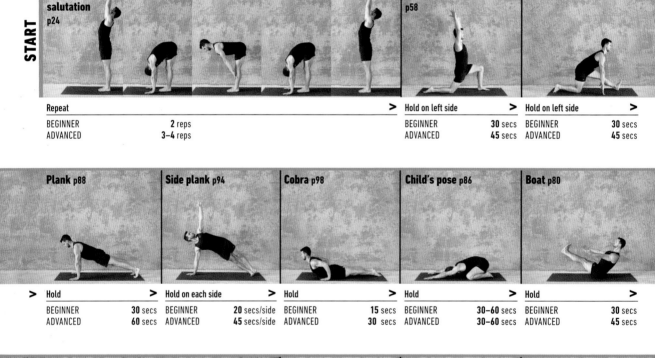

START

Half sun salutation p24

Repeat		>	**Low lunge** p58 Hold on left side	>	**Half split** p64 Hold on left side	>
BEGINNER	2 reps		BEGINNER	30 secs	BEGINNER	30 secs
ADVANCED	3–4 reps		ADVANCED	45 secs	ADVANCED	45 secs

Plank p88   **Side plank** p94   **Cobra** p98   **Child's pose** p86   **Boat** p80

> Hold	>	Hold on each side	>	Hold	>	Hold	>	Hold	>
BEGINNER	30 secs	BEGINNER	20 secs/side	BEGINNER	15 secs	BEGINNER	30–60 secs	BEGINNER	30 secs
ADVANCED	60 secs	ADVANCED	45 secs/side	ADVANCED	30 secs	ADVANCED	30–60 secs	ADVANCED	45 secs

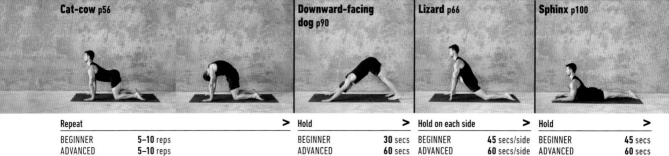

Cat-cow p56   **Downward-facing dog** p90   **Lizard** p66   **Sphinx** p100

Repeat		>	Hold	>	Hold on each side	>	Hold	>
BEGINNER	5–10 reps		BEGINNER	30 secs	BEGINNER	45 secs/side	BEGINNER	45 secs
ADVANCED	5–10 reps		ADVANCED	60 secs	ADVANCED	60 secs/side	ADVANCED	60 secs

GOOD FOR

• Workers who are on their feet at a workstation or stand-up desk

• After concerts, long walks, or other activities that involve being on your feet for hours at a time

GUIDELINES

• Hold the postures for the time given, or repeat for the reps given, breathing consciously to work deeper into the poses.

• If the instructions say to hold on each side, do the left side and then the right side in succession.

• Move as fluidly as possible from one posture to the next without resetting to a starting position unless necessary.

• This routine stretches the muscles used to stand, and strengthens those not used when standing. Although it's restorative, it's also a strength workout, so push yourself!

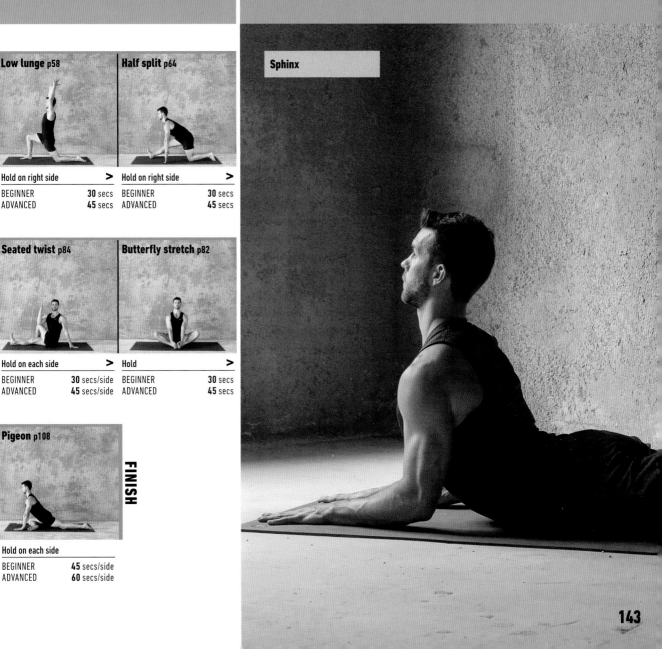

Sphinx

Low lunge p58		Half split p64	
Hold on right side	**>**	**Hold on right side**	**>**
BEGINNER	**30** secs	BEGINNER	**30** secs
ADVANCED	**45** secs	ADVANCED	**45** secs

Seated twist p84		Butterfly stretch p82	
Hold on each side	**>**	**Hold**	**>**
BEGINNER	**30** secs/side	BEGINNER	**30** secs
ADVANCED	**45** secs/side	ADVANCED	**45** secs

Pigeon p108	
Hold on each side	
BEGINNER	**45** secs/side
ADVANCED	**60** secs/side

FINISH

143

POSTURE FIXER-UPPER

Say goodbye to slouching. This is a workout you can do every morning to help you project confidence and stand tall the whole day, without having to think about it. These postures open your chest, and strengthen your core and spine, contributing to long-term posture improvement.

START

Bridge p116	Child's pose p86	Plank p88	Chair p32	High lunge p38
Hold >	Hold >	Hold >	Hold >	Hold on each side >
BEGINNER 30 secs	BEGINNER 30 secs	BEGINNER 30 secs	BEGINNER 30 secs	BEGINNER 30 secs/side
ADVANCED 60 secs	ADVANCED 60 secs	ADVANCED 60 secs	ADVANCED 60 secs	ADVANCED 60 secs/side

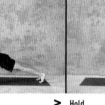

Tree p74	Airplane p68	Plank p88	Low plank p96	Cobra p98
> Hold on each side >	Hold on each side >	Hold >	Hold >	Hold >
BEGINNER 30 secs/side	BEGINNER 30 secs/side	BEGINNER 15 secs	BEGINNER 15 secs	BEGINNER 15 secs
ADVANCED 45 secs/side	ADVANCED 45 secs/side	ADVANCED 30 secs	ADVANCED 30 secs	ADVANCED 30 secs

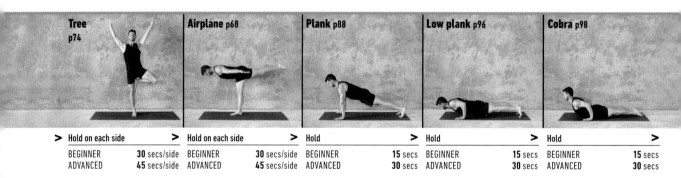

Standing backbend p28	Boat p80	Sphinx p100
Hold >	Hold >	Hold
BEGINNER 30 secs	BEGINNER 30 secs	BEGINNER 30 secs
ADVANCED 60 secs	ADVANCED 60 secs	ADVANCED 60 secs

FINISH

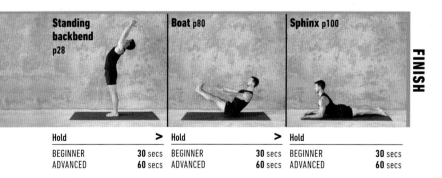

GOOD FOR

- Anyone who sits for prolonged periods
- People with chronic neck and spine pain
- Office workers and desk jockeys
- People with long commutes, frequent flyers, and anyone who drives often
- Those who spend a lot of time on their phones or tablets

GUIDELINES

- Hold the postures for the time given, breathing consciously to work deeper into the poses.
- If the instructions say to hold on each side, do the left side and then the right side in succession.
- Your body is (most likely) used to poor posture, so you'll need to push yourself slightly beyond your comfort level in order to make noticeable posture improvement.
- Constantly strive to keep the front of your torso as long as possible, from your pubic bone to sternum.

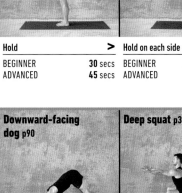

Standing backbend p28

Standing sidebend p30

Hold	>	Hold on each side	>
BEGINNER	30 secs	BEGINNER	30 secs/side
ADVANCED	45 secs	ADVANCED	45 secs/side

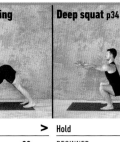

Downward-facing dog p90

Deep squat p34

Hold	>	Hold	>
BEGINNER	30 secs	BEGINNER	30 secs
ADVANCED	60 secs	ADVANCED	45 secs

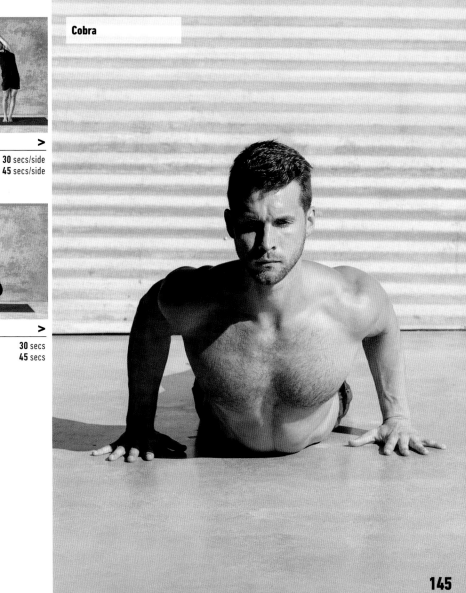

Cobra

145

STIFF NECK RELIEF

This full-body, low-intensity workout addresses the root causes of neck pain, while also immediately alleviating the symptoms. Use this routine to stretch the tight muscles in your upper back, strengthen your neck and shoulder muscles, and develop long-term, improved neck posture on a day-to-day basis.

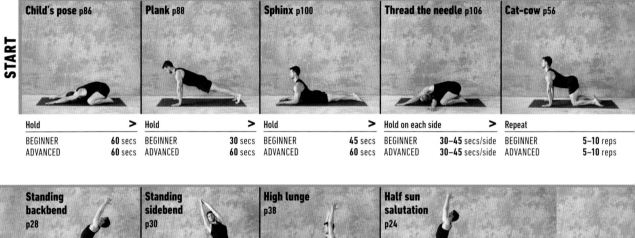

START

Child's pose p86	Plank p88	Sphinx p100	Thread the needle p106	Cat-cow p56
Hold >	Hold >	Hold >	Hold on each side >	Repeat
BEGINNER 60 secs	BEGINNER 30 secs	BEGINNER 45 secs	BEGINNER 30–45 secs/side	BEGINNER 5–10 reps
ADVANCED 60 secs	ADVANCED 60 secs	ADVANCED 60 secs	ADVANCED 30–45 secs/side	ADVANCED 5–10 reps

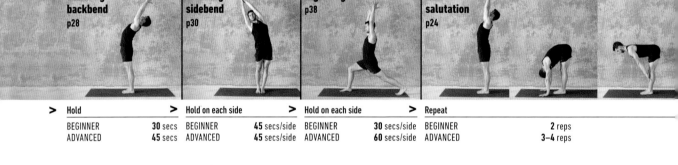

Standing backbend p28	Standing sidebend p30	High lunge p38	Half sun salutation p24	
Hold >	Hold on each side >	Hold on each side >	Repeat	
BEGINNER 30 secs	BEGINNER 45 secs/side	BEGINNER 30 secs/side	BEGINNER 2 reps	
ADVANCED 45 secs	ADVANCED 45 secs/side	ADVANCED 60 secs/side	ADVANCED 3–4 reps	

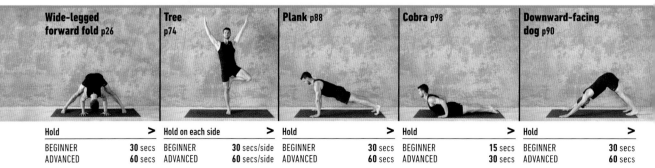

Wide-legged forward fold p26	Tree p74	Plank p88	Cobra p98	Downward-facing dog p90
Hold >	Hold on each side >	Hold >	Hold >	Hold >
BEGINNER 30 secs	BEGINNER 30 secs/side	BEGINNER 30 secs	BEGINNER 15 secs	BEGINNER 30 secs
ADVANCED 60 secs	ADVANCED 60 secs/side	ADVANCED 60 secs	ADVANCED 30 secs	ADVANCED 60 secs

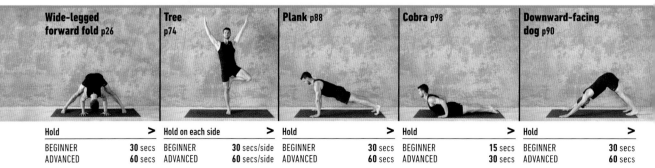

RESTORATIVE AND STRENGTHENING

GOOD FOR

- Anyone who sits for prolonged periods
- People with chronic neck and spine pain
- Those who look down at their phone or smart device often
- People who have poor posture
- Anyone who holds tension in their neck and shoulders

GUIDELINES

- Hold the postures for the time given, or repeat for the reps given, breathing consciously to work deeper into the poses.
- If the instructions say to hold on each side, do the left side and then the right side in succession.
- Maintain length in your neck. Think of pulling the crown of your head as far away from your shoulders as possible.
- Rather than letting your head fall in one direction or the other, engage your neck muscles throughout this routine to hold your head upright and actively strengthen your neck.

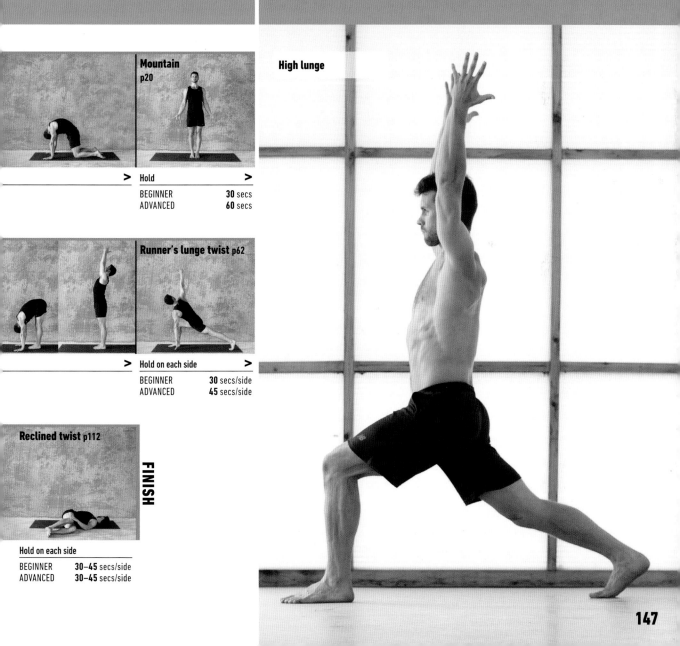

Mountain p20

> **Hold** >

BEGINNER	**30** secs
ADVANCED	**60** secs

Runner's lunge twist p62

> **Hold on each side** >

BEGINNER	**30** secs/side
ADVANCED	**45** secs/side

FINISH

Reclined twist p112

Hold on each side

BEGINNER	**30–45** secs/side
ADVANCED	**30–45** secs/side

High lunge

147

ESSENTIAL HIP MOBILITY

This workout focuses on increasing the range of motion of your hips, letting you work deeper into postures, improving your squats and lunges, and preventing injury in your knees, ankles, hips, and back. It also helps relieve pressure or tension in your lower back. Use this routine on a regular basis to keep your spine feeling great and your hips moving well.

START

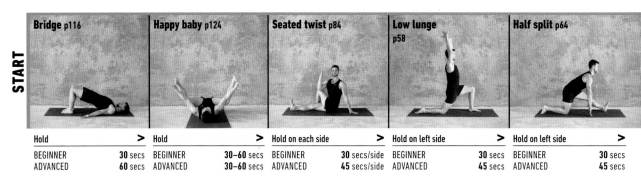

Bridge p116	**Happy baby** p124	**Seated twist** p84	**Low lunge** p58	**Half split** p64
Hold >	Hold >	Hold on each side >	Hold on left side >	Hold on left side >
BEGINNER 30 secs	BEGINNER 30–60 secs	BEGINNER 30 secs/side	BEGINNER 30 secs	BEGINNER 30 secs
ADVANCED 60 secs	ADVANCED 30–60 secs	ADVANCED 45 secs/side	ADVANCED 45 secs	ADVANCED 45 secs

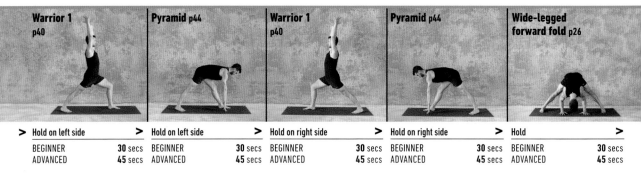

Warrior 1 p40	**Pyramid** p44	**Warrior 1** p40	**Pyramid** p44	**Wide-legged forward fold** p26
> Hold on left side >	Hold on left side >	Hold on right side >	Hold on right side >	Hold >
BEGINNER 30 secs	BEGINNER 30 secs	BEGINNER 30 secs	BEGINNER 30 secs	BEGINNER 30 secs
ADVANCED 45 secs	ADVANCED 45 secs	ADVANCED 45 secs	ADVANCED 45 secs	ADVANCED 45 secs

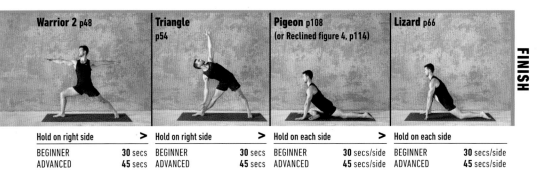

FINISH

Warrior 2 p48	**Triangle** p54	**Pigeon** p108 (or Reclined figure 4, p114)	**Lizard** p66
Hold on right side >	Hold on right side >	Hold on each side >	Hold on each side
BEGINNER 30 secs	BEGINNER 30 secs	BEGINNER 30 secs/side	BEGINNER 30 secs/side
ADVANCED 45 secs	ADVANCED 45 secs	ADVANCED 45 secs/side	ADVANCED 45 secs/side

GOOD FOR

- Anyone with a stiff lower back
- People who sit for prolonged periods
- Inactive people
- Athletes who need injury-resistant ankles and knees

GUIDELINES

- Hold the postures for the time given, breathing consciously to work deeper into the poses.
- If the instructions say to hold on each side, do the left side and then the right side in succession.
- Move as fluidly as possible from one posture to the next without resetting to a starting position unless necessary.
- If you're not used to working on hip mobility, it will likely be difficult at first. Keep at it and stay consistent.

Low lunge p58	Half split p64
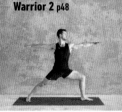	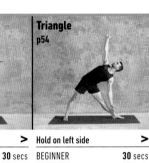
Hold on right side >	**Hold on right side** >
BEGINNER **30** secs	BEGINNER **30** secs
ADVANCED **45** secs	ADVANCED **45** secs

Warrior 2 p48	Triangle p54
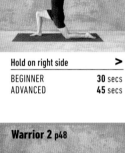	
Hold on left side >	**Hold on left side** >
BEGINNER **30** secs	BEGINNER **30** secs
ADVANCED **45** secs	ADVANCED **45** secs

Triangle

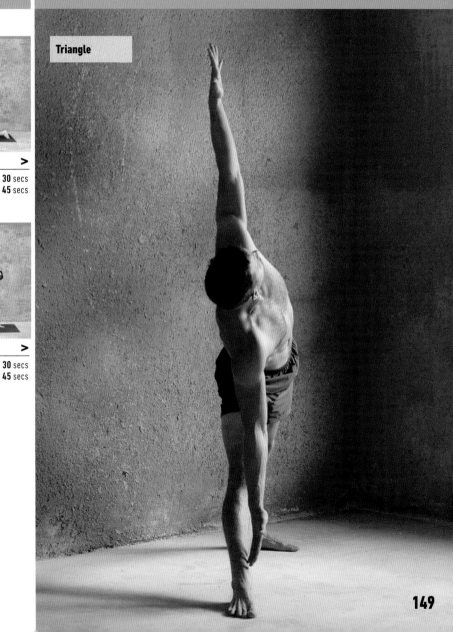

TOTAL-BODY STRENGTH

Ready to be challenged? This full-length workout strengthens the entire body with the most difficult postures in this book. Build and tone muscle in your body from head to toe, while simultaneously improving mobility in the hips, shoulders, ankles, and spine.

START

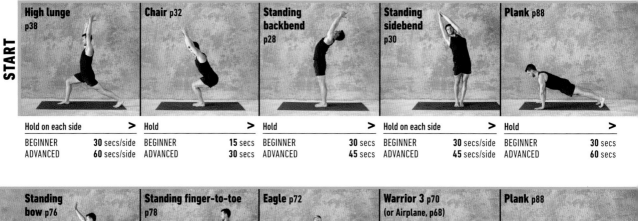

High lunge p38

Hold on each side	>
BEGINNER	30 secs/side
ADVANCED	60 secs/side

Chair p32

Hold	>
BEGINNER	15 secs
ADVANCED	30 secs

Standing backbend p28

Hold	>
BEGINNER	30 secs
ADVANCED	45 secs

Standing sidebend p30

Hold on each side	>
BEGINNER	30 secs/side
ADVANCED	45 secs/side

Plank p88

Hold	>
BEGINNER	30 secs
ADVANCED	60 secs

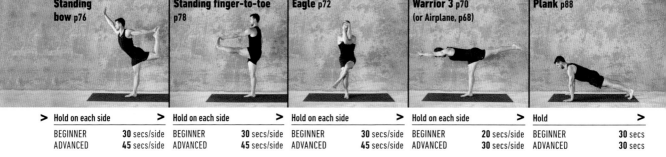

Standing bow p76

>	Hold on each side	>
	BEGINNER	30 secs/side
	ADVANCED	45 secs/side

Standing finger-to-toe p78

Hold on each side	>
BEGINNER	30 secs/side
ADVANCED	45 secs/side

Eagle p72

Hold on each side	>
BEGINNER	30 secs/side
ADVANCED	45 secs/side

Warrior 3 p70 (or Airplane, p68)

Hold on each side	>
BEGINNER	20 secs/side
ADVANCED	30 secs/side

Plank p88

Hold	>
BEGINNER	30 secs
ADVANCED	30 secs

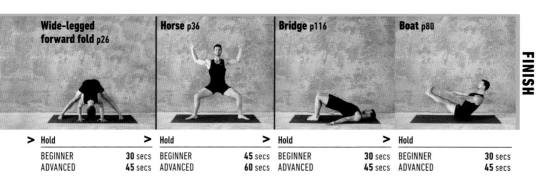

Wide-legged forward fold p26

>	Hold	>
	BEGINNER	30 secs
	ADVANCED	45 secs

Horse p36

Hold	>
BEGINNER	45 secs
ADVANCED	60 secs

Bridge p116

Hold	>
BEGINNER	30 secs
ADVANCED	45 secs

Boat p80

Hold
BEGINNER 30 secs
ADVANCED 45 secs

FINISH

GOOD FOR

• People who want to build muscle and increase muscle tone

• Anyone looking for a challenging bodyweight or yoga workout

• Athletes who want to replace a day of resistance training with a yoga workout

GUIDELINES

• Hold the postures for the time given, breathing consciously to work deeper into the poses.

• If the instructions say to hold on each side, do the left side and then the right side in succession.

• This is meant to be a challenge, so don't give up on your first (or even 100th) try. Keep breathing, relax your body, and you'll make it through. Take a break if you need to, but set a goal to get through the entire routine without stopping.

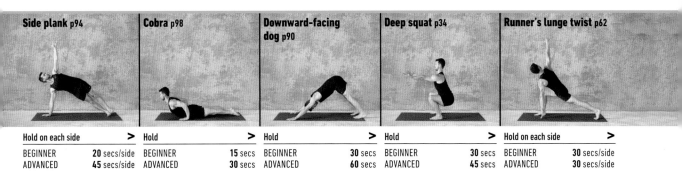

Side plank p94		Cobra p98		Downward-facing dog p90		Deep squat p34		Runner's lunge twist p62	
Hold on each side	**>**	**Hold**	**>**	**Hold**	**>**	**Hold**	**>**	**Hold on each side**	**>**
BEGINNER	**20** secs/side	BEGINNER	**15** secs	BEGINNER	**30** secs	BEGINNER	**30** secs	BEGINNER	**30** secs/side
ADVANCED	**45** secs/side	ADVANCED	**30** secs	ADVANCED	**60** secs	ADVANCED	**45** secs	ADVANCED	**30** secs/side

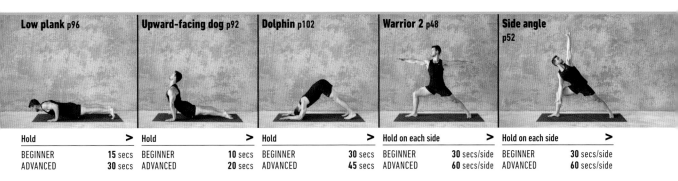

Low plank p96		Upward-facing dog p92		Dolphin p102		Warrior 2 p48		Side angle p52	
Hold	**>**	**Hold**	**>**	**Hold**	**>**	**Hold on each side**	**>**	**Hold on each side**	**>**
BEGINNER	**15** secs	BEGINNER	**10** secs	BEGINNER	**30** secs	BEGINNER	**30** secs/side	BEGINNER	**30** secs/side
ADVANCED	**30** secs	ADVANCED	**20** secs	ADVANCED	**45** secs	ADVANCED	**60** secs/side	ADVANCED	**60** secs/side

TOO MUCH SITTING

Stand up to your desk-bound life and kick the negative effects to the curb. Frequent sitting, whether at a desk, in your car, or on the couch, causes weakness, muscle imbalances, tightness, and poor posture. This routine strengthens the weaknesses, stretches the tight areas, and corrects the imbalances to restore good posture. Use this routine regularly if you sit a lot!

START

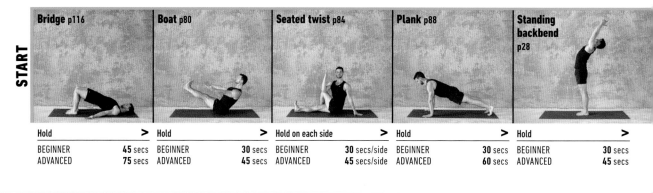

Bridge p116	Boat p80	Seated twist p84	Plank p88	Standing backbend p28
Hold >	Hold >	Hold on each side >	Hold >	Hold >
BEGINNER 45 secs	BEGINNER 30 secs	BEGINNER 30 secs/side	BEGINNER 30 secs	BEGINNER 30 secs
ADVANCED 75 secs	ADVANCED 45 secs	ADVANCED 45 secs/side	ADVANCED 60 secs	ADVANCED 45 secs

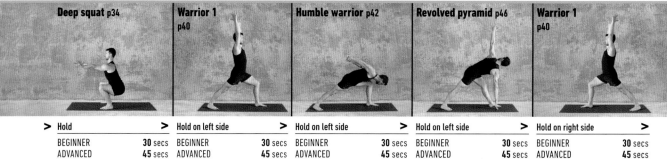

Deep squat p34	Warrior 1 p40	Humble warrior p42	Revolved pyramid p46	Warrior 1 p40
> Hold >	Hold on left side >	Hold on left side >	Hold on left side >	Hold on right side >
BEGINNER 30 secs	BEGINNER 30 secs	BEGINNER 30 secs	BEGINNER 30 secs	BEGINNER 30 secs
ADVANCED 45 secs	ADVANCED 45 secs	ADVANCED 45 secs	ADVANCED 45 secs	ADVANCED 45 secs

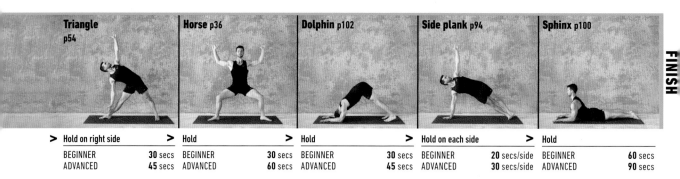

Triangle p54	Horse p36	Dolphin p102	Side plank p94	Sphinx p100
> Hold on right side >	Hold >	Hold >	Hold on each side >	Hold
BEGINNER 30 secs	BEGINNER 30 secs	BEGINNER 30 secs	BEGINNER 20 secs/side	BEGINNER 60 secs
ADVANCED 45 secs	ADVANCED 60 secs	ADVANCED 45 secs	ADVANCED 30 secs/side	ADVANCED 90 secs

FINISH

GOOD FOR

- Anyone who sits for prolonged periods
- Athletes who want to strengthen their core
- People who want to improve posture

GUIDELINES

- Hold the postures for the time given, breathing consciously to work deeper into the poses.
- If the instructions say to hold on each side, do the left side and then the right side in succession.
- Move as fluidly as possible from one posture to the next without resetting to a starting position unless necessary.
- Sitting is particularly bad for your core, so focus on that area from your mid-thighs up to your sternum (on the front, back, and sides) as you do this routine.

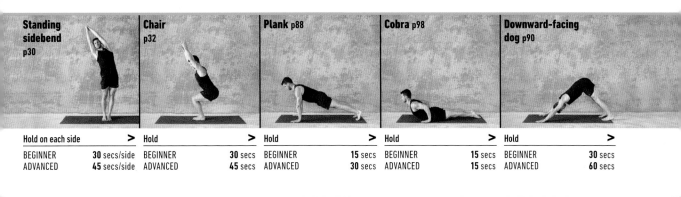

Standing sidebend p30

Hold on each side	>
BEGINNER	30 secs/side
ADVANCED	45 secs/side

Chair p32

Hold	>
BEGINNER	30 secs
ADVANCED	45 secs

Plank p88

Hold	>
BEGINNER	15 secs
ADVANCED	30 secs

Cobra p98

Hold	>
BEGINNER	15 secs
ADVANCED	15 secs

Downward-facing dog p90

Hold	>
BEGINNER	30 secs
ADVANCED	60 secs

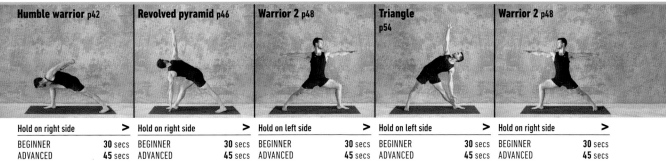

Humble warrior p42

Hold on right side	>
BEGINNER	30 secs
ADVANCED	45 secs

Revolved pyramid p46

Hold on right side	>
BEGINNER	30 secs
ADVANCED	45 secs

Warrior 2 p48

Hold on left side	>
BEGINNER	30 secs
ADVANCED	45 secs

Triangle p54

Hold on left side	>
BEGINNER	30 secs
ADVANCED	45 secs

Warrior 2 p48

Hold on right side	>
BEGINNER	30 secs
ADVANCED	45 secs

STRENGTHENING

ENDURANCE FOR STANDING

If you stand often, you need to strengthen the muscles
that keep you upright and support good posture. Use this
routine to build endurance and strength in your spine, core,
glutes, hips, and shoulders so that you can avoid fatigue and
stand as long as you need to without thinking twice.

START

High lunge p38	Chair p32	Tree p74	Airplane p68	Standing bow p76
Hold on each side	**Hold**	**Hold on each side**	**Hold on each side**	**Hold on each side**
BEGINNER 30 secs/side	BEGINNER 30 secs	BEGINNER 30 secs/side	BEGINNER 30 secs/side	BEGINNER 30 secs/side
ADVANCED 60 secs/side	ADVANCED 45 secs	ADVANCED 45 secs/side	ADVANCED 45 secs/side	ADVANCED 45 secs/side

   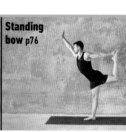

Eagle p72	Deep squat p34	Wide-legged forward fold p26	Warrior 2 p48	Horse p36
Hold on each side	**Hold**	**Hold**	**Hold on each side**	**Hold**
BEGINNER 30 secs/side	BEGINNER 30 secs	BEGINNER 30 secs	BEGINNER 30 secs/side	BEGINNER 30 secs
ADVANCED 45 secs/side	ADVANCED 45 secs	ADVANCED 45 secs	ADVANCED 45 secs/side	ADVANCED 60 secs

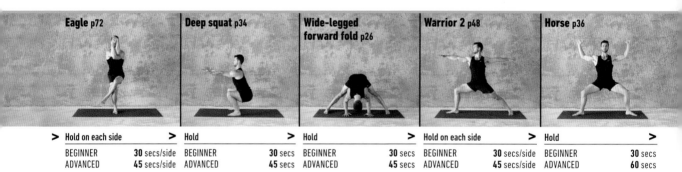

FINISH

Dolphin p102	Full locust p104	Child's pose p86 (optional)
Hold	**Hold**	**Hold**
BEGINNER 30 secs	BEGINNER 20 secs	BEGINNER 30–60 secs
ADVANCED 45 secs	ADVANCED 30 secs	ADVANCED 30–60 secs

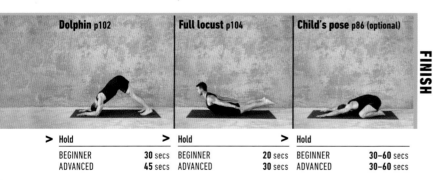

154

GOOD FOR

- People who want to have improved posture while standing

- Fitness enthusiasts and athletes who want to improve body awareness and muscle activation

GUIDELINES

- Hold the postures for the time given, breathing consciously to work deeper into the poses.

- If the instructions say to hold on each side, do the left side and then the right side in succession.

- This routine engages the correct muscles for standing, so be mindful of where you feel engagement and use those muscles when standing.

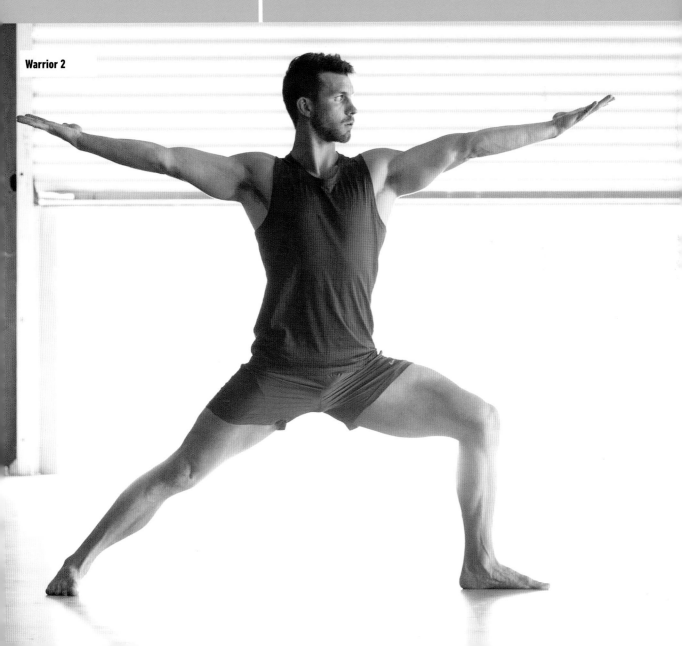

Warrior 2

FOUNDATIONAL CORE STRENGTH

Your core is more than just abs. Use this routine to strengthen every part of the core, and you'll get better at everything you physically do. This comprehensive workout develops mastery of all the core muscles from your mid-thighs to sternum, for strong, pain-free movement in your daily activity. These postures build the strength you need to move well and prevent injury.

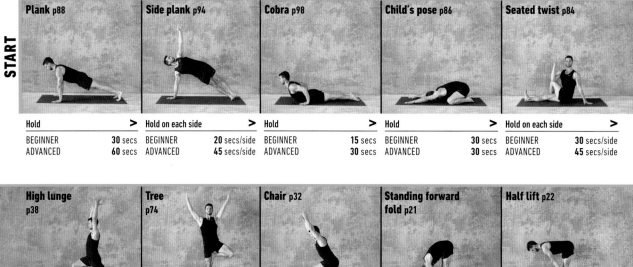

START

Plank p88
Hold >
BEGINNER 30 secs
ADVANCED 60 secs

Side plank p94
Hold on each side >
BEGINNER 20 secs/side
ADVANCED 45 secs/side

Cobra p98
Hold >
BEGINNER 15 secs
ADVANCED 30 secs

Child's pose p86
Hold >
BEGINNER 30 secs
ADVANCED 30 secs

Seated twist p84
Hold on each side >
BEGINNER 30 secs/side
ADVANCED 45 secs/side

High lunge p38
> Hold on each side >
BEGINNER 30 secs/side
ADVANCED 60 secs/side

Tree p74
Hold on each side >
BEGINNER 30 secs/side
ADVANCED 60 secs/side

Chair p32
Hold >
BEGINNER 30 secs
ADVANCED 45 secs

Standing forward fold p21
Hold >
BEGINNER 15 secs
ADVANCED 15 secs

Half lift p22
Hold >
BEGINNER 15 secs
ADVANCED 15 secs

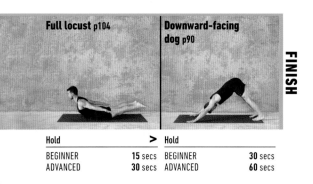

Full locust p104
Hold >
BEGINNER 15 secs
ADVANCED 30 secs

Downward-facing dog p90
Hold
BEGINNER 30 secs
ADVANCED 60 secs

FINISH

GOOD FOR

- Beginners new to yoga or people new to fitness in general
- Active people who haven't done core-focused workouts before
- People recovering from back injury
- Athletes with back pain
- Anyone prone to injuries of any type

GUIDELINES

- Hold the postures for the time given, breathing consciously to work deeper into the poses.
- If the instructions say to hold on each side, do the left side and then the right side in succession.
- Focus on the proper engagement in the mid-section of your body in every posture.

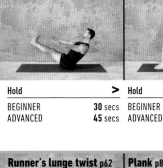

Boat p80

Hold	>
BEGINNER	**30** secs
ADVANCED	**45** secs

Bridge p116

Hold	>
BEGINNER	**30** secs
ADVANCED	**45** secs

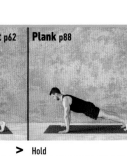

Runner's lunge twist p62

Hold on each side	>
BEGINNER	**30** secs/side
ADVANCED	**30** secs/side

Plank p88

Hold	>
BEGINNER	**30** secs
ADVANCED	**60** secs

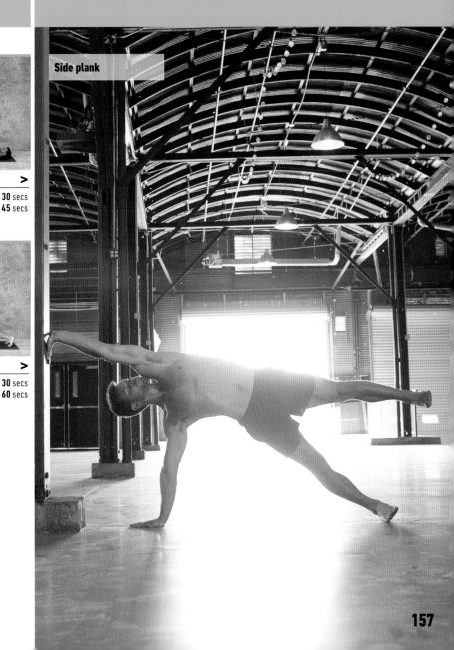

Side plank

ABS ON FIRE

Get ready to work! This ab-focused routine strengthens not only your core and spine, but the rest of your body, too. Consciously engage the core for every part of this workout so that you build a strong body from the inside out. Be sure to maintain proper technique and control for every posture to avoid expending energy on poor form—or worse, risk injury.

START

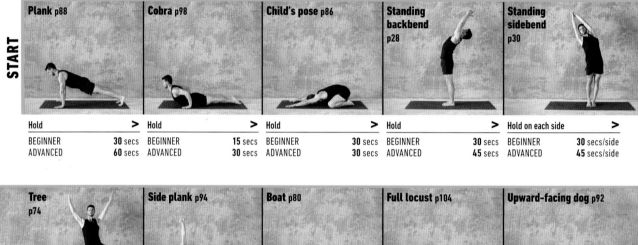

Plank p88

Hold	>
BEGINNER	30 secs
ADVANCED	60 secs

Cobra p98

Hold	>
BEGINNER	15 secs
ADVANCED	30 secs

Child's pose p86

Hold	>
BEGINNER	30 secs
ADVANCED	30 secs

Standing backbend p28

Hold	>
BEGINNER	30 secs
ADVANCED	45 secs

Standing sidebend p30

Hold on each side	>
BEGINNER	30 secs/side
ADVANCED	45 secs/side

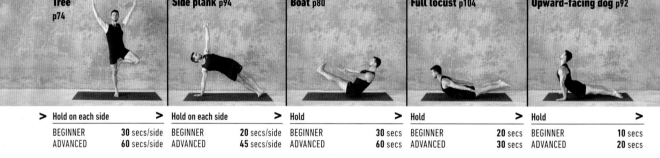

Tree p74

> Hold on each side >	
BEGINNER	30 secs/side
ADVANCED	60 secs/side

Side plank p94

Hold on each side	>
BEGINNER	20 secs/side
ADVANCED	45 secs/side

Boat p80

Hold	>
BEGINNER	30 secs
ADVANCED	60 secs

Full locust p104

Hold	>
BEGINNER	20 secs
ADVANCED	30 secs

Upward-facing dog p92

Hold	>
BEGINNER	10 secs
ADVANCED	20 secs

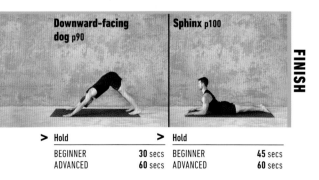

FINISH

Downward-facing dog p90

> Hold >	
BEGINNER	30 secs
ADVANCED	60 secs

Sphinx p100

Hold	
BEGINNER	45 secs
ADVANCED	60 secs

GOOD FOR

• Athletes and fitness enthusiasts who want to significantly increase core strength

• People who have consistent back pain during exercise

• Anyone who wants to prevent injury in the spine, hips, and knees

• Busy people pressed for time who need a quick, effective workout

GUIDELINES

• Hold the postures for the time given, breathing consciously to work deeper into the poses.

• If the instructions say to hold on each side, do the left side and then the right side in succession.

• Keep your breathing slow and controlled.

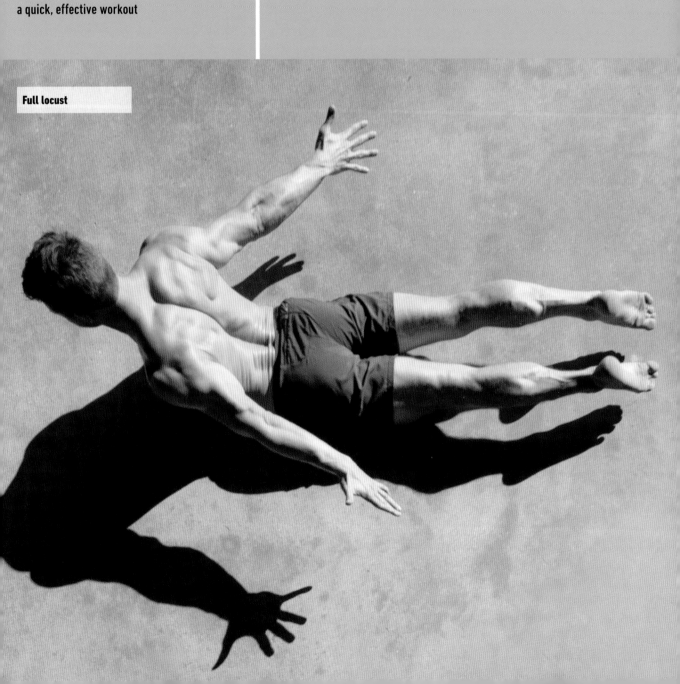

Full locust

STRONG SPINE, STRONG BODY

Twist, bend, and arch for a strong back. Most people are sedentary with stiff and inflexible backs. By strengthening the muscles connected to your spine and stretching the hips, this workout addresses the root causes of back pain and improves spinal mobility. Move the spine in every direction possible with these postures to improve range of motion.

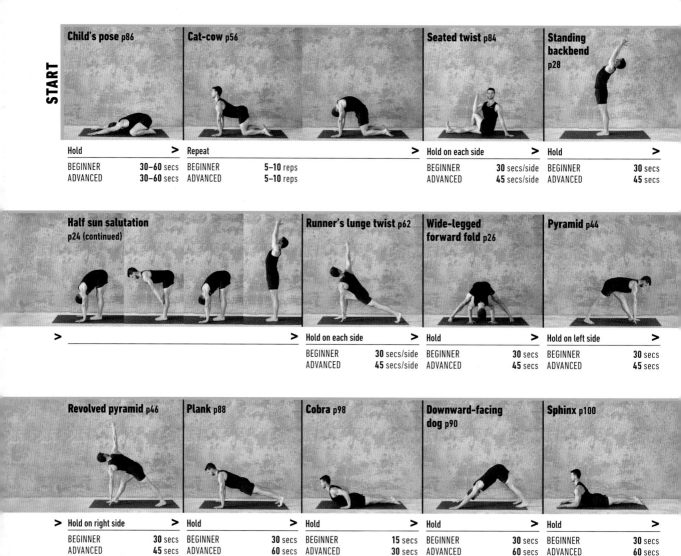

START

STRENGTHENING

Child's pose p86

Hold	>
BEGINNER	30–60 secs
ADVANCED	30–60 secs

Cat-cow p56

Repeat		>
BEGINNER	5–10 reps	
ADVANCED	5–10 reps	

Seated twist p84

Hold on each side	>
BEGINNER	30 secs/side
ADVANCED	45 secs/side

Standing backbend p28

Hold	>
BEGINNER	30 secs
ADVANCED	45 secs

Half sun salutation p24 (continued)

> _____ >

Runner's lunge twist p62

Hold on each side	>
BEGINNER	30 secs/side
ADVANCED	45 secs/side

Wide-legged forward fold p26

Hold	>
BEGINNER	30 secs
ADVANCED	45 secs

Pyramid p44

Hold on left side	>
BEGINNER	30 secs
ADVANCED	45 secs

Revolved pyramid p46

> Hold on right side	>
BEGINNER	30 secs
ADVANCED	45 secs

Plank p88

Hold	>
BEGINNER	30 secs
ADVANCED	60 secs

Cobra p98

Hold	>
BEGINNER	15 secs
ADVANCED	30 secs

Downward-facing dog p90

Hold	>
BEGINNER	30 secs
ADVANCED	60 secs

Sphinx p100

Hold	>
BEGINNER	30 secs
ADVANCED	60 secs

160

GOOD FOR

- Athletes and fitness enthusiasts hoping to prevent spinal injury
- Anyone with back pain
- People who don't move their spine through its full range of motion on a regular basis
- Maintaining spinal mobility for everyday functions such as driving, bending over, and turning your head

GUIDELINES

- Hold the postures for the time given, or repeat for the reps given, breathing consciously to work deeper into the poses.
- If the instructions say to hold on each side, do the left side and then the right side in succession.
- Move as fluidly as possible from one posture to the next without resetting to a starting position unless necessary.
- For every one of these postures, make sure to lengthen the spine first in order to bend deeper, twist further, or arch more.

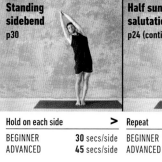

Standing sidebend p30

Half sun salutation p24 (continues)

Hold on each side	>	Repeat	>
BEGINNER	**30** secs/side	BEGINNER	**1–2** reps
ADVANCED	**45** secs/side	ADVANCED	**2–3** reps

Revolved pyramid p46

Pyramid p44

Hold on left side	>	Hold on right side	>
BEGINNER	**30** secs	BEGINNER	**30** secs
ADVANCED	**45** secs	ADVANCED	**45** secs

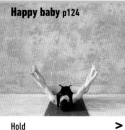

Happy baby p124

Reclined twist p112

Hold	>	Hold on each side	
BEGINNER	**30–60** secs	BEGINNER	**30–45** secs/side
ADVANCED	**30–60** secs	ADVANCED	**30–45** secs/side

FINISH

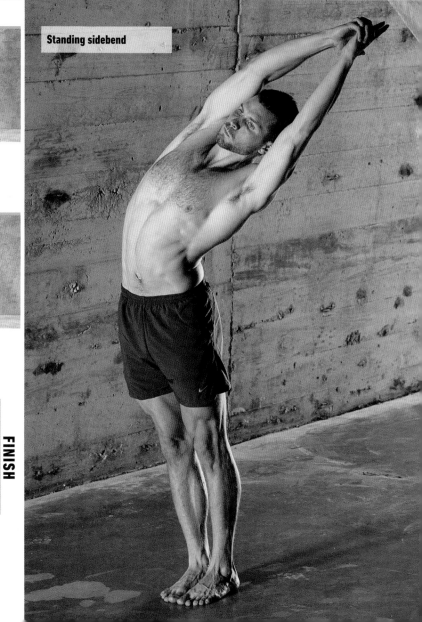

Standing sidebend

BASIC SHOULDER STRENGTH
AND MOBILITY

Prevent clicking, popping, and grinding sensations in your shoulders caused by weakness and tightness. This workout starts with warm-up postures, moves on to more intense strength work, and finishes with restorative stretches. This is the beginner's foundation for strong, injury-free shoulders.

START

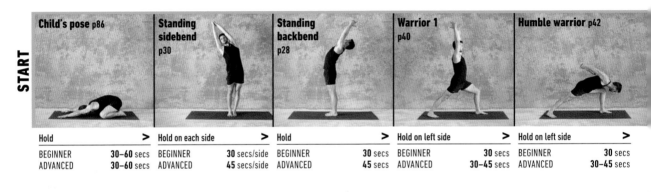

Child's pose p86		Standing sidebend p30		Standing backbend p28		Warrior 1 p40		Humble warrior p42	
Hold	>	**Hold on each side**	>	**Hold**	>	**Hold on left side**	>	**Hold on left side**	>
BEGINNER	30–60 secs	BEGINNER	30 secs/side	BEGINNER	30 secs	BEGINNER	30 secs	BEGINNER	30 secs
ADVANCED	30–60 secs	ADVANCED	45 secs/side	ADVANCED	45 secs	ADVANCED	30–45 secs	ADVANCED	30–45 secs

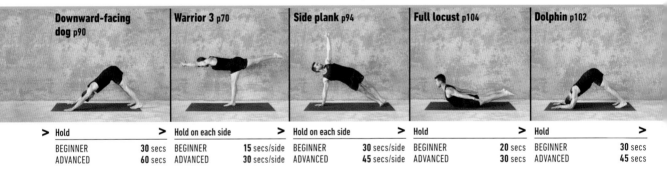

Downward-facing dog p90		Warrior 3 p70		Side plank p94		Full locust p104		Dolphin p102	
> **Hold**	>	**Hold on each side**	>	**Hold on each side**	>	**Hold**	>	**Hold**	>
BEGINNER	30 secs	BEGINNER	15 secs/side	BEGINNER	30 secs/side	BEGINNER	20 secs	BEGINNER	30 secs
ADVANCED	60 secs	ADVANCED	30 secs/side	ADVANCED	45 secs/side	ADVANCED	30 secs	ADVANCED	45 secs

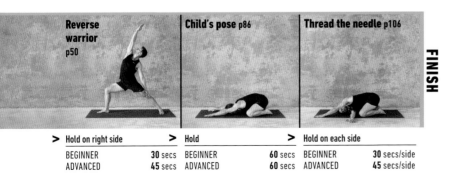

FINISH

Reverse warrior p50		Child's pose p86		Thread the needle p106	
> **Hold on right side**	>	**Hold**	>	**Hold on each side**	
BEGINNER	30 secs	BEGINNER	60 secs	BEGINNER	30 secs/side
ADVANCED	45 secs	ADVANCED	60 secs	ADVANCED	45 secs/side

GOOD FOR

- Athletes who require shoulder mobility
- Anyone with weak posture
- People recovering from rotator cuff injury
- Weight lifters who don't stretch enough
- Anyone who uses overhead motions, such as swinging or throwing

GUIDELINES

- Hold the postures for the time given, or repeat for the reps given, breathing consciously to work deeper into the poses.
- If the instructions say to hold on each side, do the left side and then the right side in succession.
- Move as fluidly as possible from one posture to the next without resetting to a starting position unless necessary.
- Challenge your strength by holding the posture for the full time, and challenge your mobility by pushing past your comfort zone—while maintaining good form, of course.

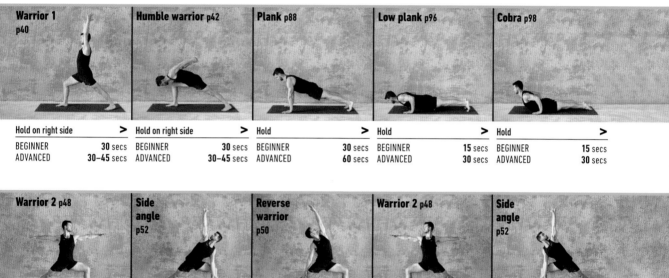

Warrior 1 p40		Humble warrior p42		Plank p88		Low plank p96		Cobra p98	
Hold on right side	>	Hold on right side	>	Hold	>	Hold	>	Hold	>
BEGINNER	30 secs	BEGINNER	30 secs	BEGINNER	30 secs	BEGINNER	15 secs	BEGINNER	15 secs
ADVANCED	30–45 secs	ADVANCED	30–45 secs	ADVANCED	60 secs	ADVANCED	30 secs	ADVANCED	30 secs

Warrior 2 p48		Side angle p52		Reverse warrior p50		Warrior 2 p48		Side angle p52	
Hold on left side	>	Hold on left side	>	Hold on left side	>	Hold on right side	>	Hold on right side	>
BEGINNER	30 secs	BEGINNER	30 secs	BEGINNER	30 secs	BEGINNER	30 secs	BEGINNER	30 secs
ADVANCED	30 secs	ADVANCED	45 secs	ADVANCED	45 secs	ADVANCED	30 secs	ADVANCED	45 secs

ADVANCED UPPER-BODY WORK
FOR BULLETPROOF SHOULDERS

These demanding postures use your whole upper body to improve the strength of your shoulders, chest, and upper back, while also improving flexibility and making you more injury-resistant. This workout makes your muscles burn, improves your shoulder endurance, and tones your upper-body physique.

START

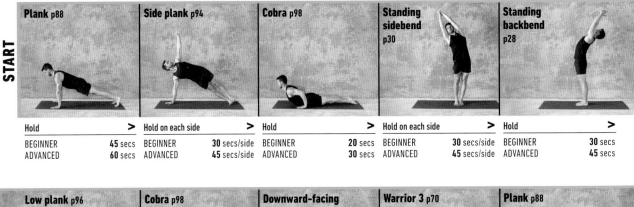

Plank p88	Side plank p94	Cobra p98	Standing sidebend p30	Standing backbend p28
Hold >	Hold on each side >	Hold >	Hold on each side >	Hold >
BEGINNER 45 secs	BEGINNER 30 secs/side	BEGINNER 20 secs	BEGINNER 30 secs/side	BEGINNER 30 secs
ADVANCED 60 secs	ADVANCED 45 secs/side	ADVANCED 30 secs	ADVANCED 45 secs/side	ADVANCED 45 secs

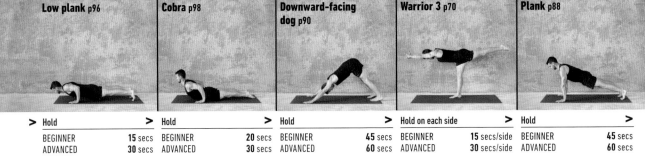

Low plank p96	Cobra p98	Downward-facing dog p90	Warrior 3 p70	Plank p88
> Hold >	Hold >	Hold >	Hold on each side >	Hold >
BEGINNER 15 secs	BEGINNER 20 secs	BEGINNER 45 secs	BEGINNER 15 secs/side	BEGINNER 45 secs
ADVANCED 30 secs	ADVANCED 30 secs	ADVANCED 60 secs	ADVANCED 30 secs/side	ADVANCED 60 secs

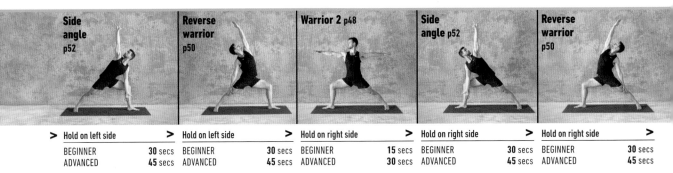

Side angle p52	Reverse warrior p50	Warrior 2 p48	Side angle p52	Reverse warrior p50
> Hold on left side >	Hold on left side >	Hold on right side >	Hold on right side >	Hold on right side >
BEGINNER 30 secs	BEGINNER 30 secs	BEGINNER 15 secs	BEGINNER 30 secs	BEGINNER 30 secs
ADVANCED 45 secs	ADVANCED 45 secs	ADVANCED 30 secs	ADVANCED 45 secs	ADVANCED 45 secs

GOOD FOR

- Athletes, swimmers, and fitness enthusiasts who want to significantly strengthen shoulders
- Those who want to develop upper-body strength for arm balances or inversions
- Weight lifters who want to prevent injury and lift more with their upper bodies
- Anyone who uses repetitive overhead motions, such as swinging or throwing

GUIDELINES

- Hold the postures for the time given, or repeat for the reps given, breathing consciously to work deeper into the poses.
- If the instructions say to hold on each side, do the left side and then the right side in succession.
- Move as fluidly as possible from one posture to the next without resetting to a starting position unless necessary.
- This routine is challenging and effective, but it can also be damaging if you push yourself with poor form. If you can't maintain proper technique, take a break.

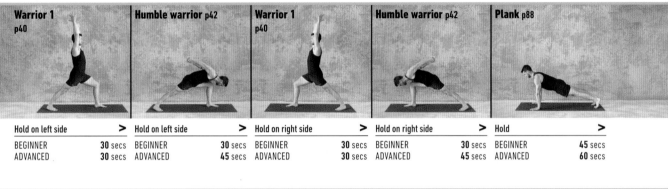

Warrior 1 p40		**Humble warrior** p42		**Warrior 1** p40		**Humble warrior** p42		**Plank** p88	
Hold on left side	>	Hold on left side	>	Hold on right side	>	Hold on right side	>	Hold	>
BEGINNER	30 secs	BEGINNER	30 secs	BEGINNER	30 secs	BEGINNER	30 secs	BEGINNER	45 secs
ADVANCED	30 secs	ADVANCED	45 secs	ADVANCED	30 secs	ADVANCED	45 secs	ADVANCED	60 secs

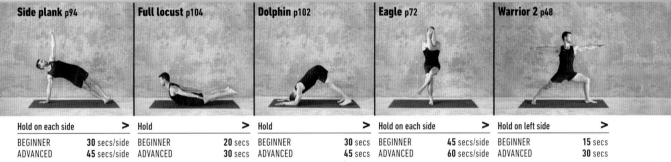

Side plank p94		**Full locust** p104		**Dolphin** p102		**Eagle** p72		**Warrior 2** p48	
Hold on each side	>	Hold	>	Hold	>	Hold on each side	>	Hold on left side	>
BEGINNER	30 secs/side	BEGINNER	20 secs	BEGINNER	30 secs	BEGINNER	45 secs/side	BEGINNER	15 secs
ADVANCED	45 secs/side	ADVANCED	30 secs	ADVANCED	45 secs	ADVANCED	60 secs/side	ADVANCED	30 secs

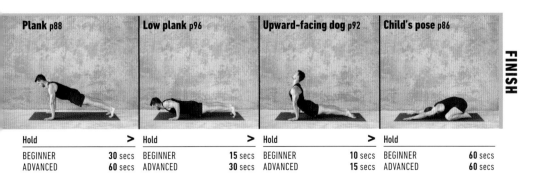

Plank p88		**Low plank** p96		**Upward-facing dog** p92		**Child's pose** p86		FINISH
Hold	>	Hold	>	Hold	>	Hold		
BEGINNER	30 secs	BEGINNER	15 secs	BEGINNER	10 secs	BEGINNER	60 secs	
ADVANCED	60 secs	ADVANCED	30 secs	ADVANCED	15 secs	ADVANCED	60 secs	

HIP STRENGTH AND MOBILITY
ESSENTIALS

These basic postures are essential for strong, healthy, and injury-resistant hips. By strengthening your hip flexors, thighs, glutes, and abdomen, you address the root cause of back pain; prevent injury in the hips, knees, and spine; and improve overall mobility and functional movement.

START

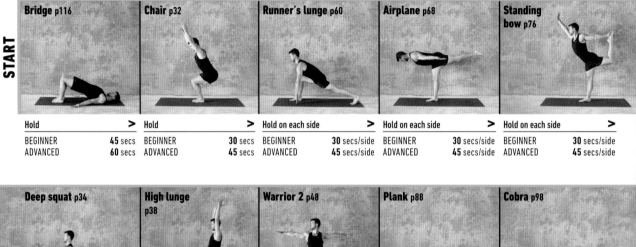

Bridge p116

Hold >

BEGINNER	45 secs
ADVANCED	60 secs

Chair p32

Hold >

BEGINNER	30 secs
ADVANCED	45 secs

Runner's lunge p60

Hold on each side >

BEGINNER	30 secs/side
ADVANCED	45 secs/side

Airplane p68

Hold on each side >

BEGINNER	30 secs/side
ADVANCED	45 secs/side

Standing bow p76

Hold on each side >

BEGINNER	30 secs/side
ADVANCED	45 secs/side

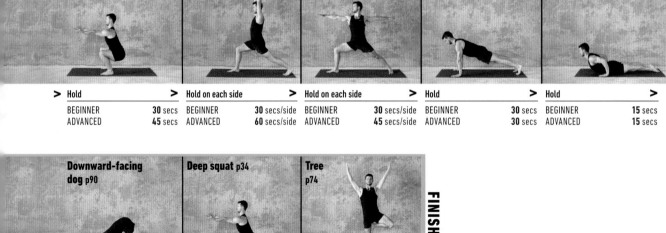

Deep squat p34

> Hold >

BEGINNER	30 secs
ADVANCED	45 secs

High lunge p38

Hold on each side >

BEGINNER	30 secs/side
ADVANCED	60 secs/side

Warrior 2 p48

Hold on each side >

BEGINNER	30 secs/side
ADVANCED	45 secs/side

Plank p88

Hold >

BEGINNER	30 secs
ADVANCED	30 secs

Cobra p98

Hold >

BEGINNER	15 secs
ADVANCED	15 secs

Downward-facing dog p90

> Hold >

BEGINNER	30 secs
ADVANCED	60 secs

Deep squat p34

Hold >

BEGINNER	30 secs
ADVANCED	60 secs

Tree p74

Hold on each side

BEGINNER	30 secs/side
ADVANCED	60 secs/side

FINISH

166

GOOD FOR

- People with back or knee problems
- Anyone who sits for prolonged periods
- Those who have never done yoga, pilates, or other similar core-focused workouts

GUIDELINES

- Hold the postures for the time given, breathing consciously to work deeper into the poses.
- If the instructions say to hold on each side, do the left side and then the right side in succession.
- This is all about the hips, so take time to focus on what you should be doing with your hips in each posture. Pay close attention to minor details, and how making small tweaks creates significant changes—that's how you get stronger.

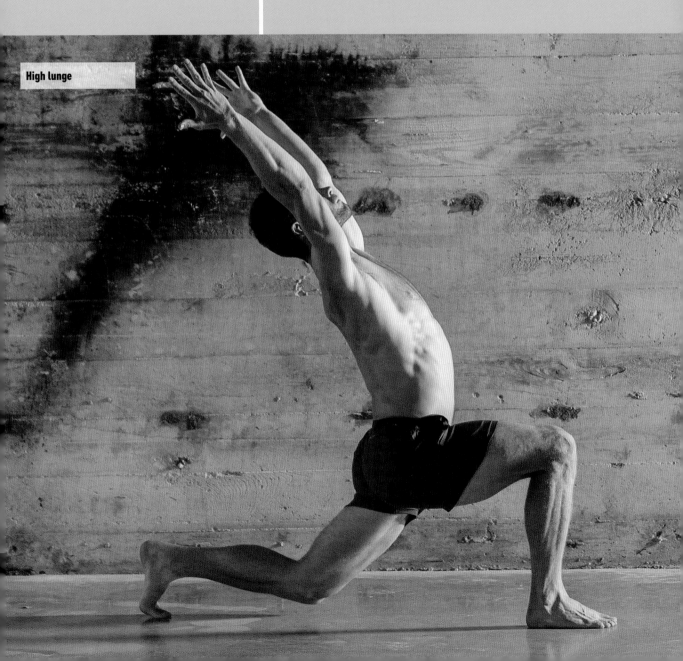

High lunge

STRONG HIPS CHALLENGE

If you're ready for a significant but rewarding challenge, this advanced workout is for you. Skip leg day at the gym, and do this sequence instead. This collection of challenging postures builds hip strength, endurance, and mobility, while also improving balance. You will work one leg at a time for an extra burn.

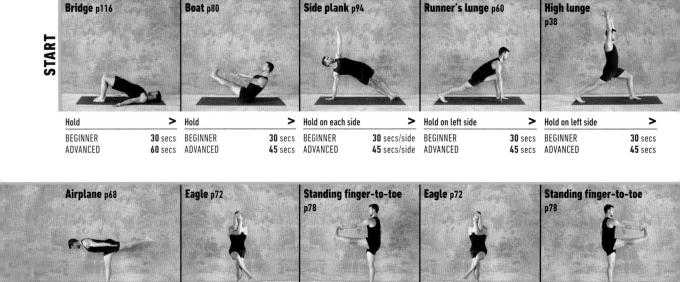

START

Bridge p116	Boat p80	Side plank p94	Runner's lunge p60	High lunge p38
Hold >	Hold >	Hold on each side >	Hold on left side >	Hold on left side >
BEGINNER 30 secs	BEGINNER 30 secs	BEGINNER 30 secs/side	BEGINNER 30 secs	BEGINNER 30 secs
ADVANCED 60 secs	ADVANCED 45 secs	ADVANCED 45 secs/side	ADVANCED 45 secs	ADVANCED 45 secs

Airplane p68	Eagle p72	Standing finger-to-toe p78	Eagle p72	Standing finger-to-toe p78
> Hold on right side >	Hold on left side >	Hold on left side >	Hold on right side >	Hold on right side >
BEGINNER 30 secs/side	BEGINNER 30 secs	BEGINNER 30 secs	BEGINNER 30 secs	BEGINNER 30 secs
ADVANCED 45 secs/side	ADVANCED 45 secs	ADVANCED 45 secs	ADVANCED 45 secs	ADVANCED 45 secs

Side angle p52	Reverse warrior p50	Tree p74	Downward-facing dog p90	Deep squat p34
> Hold on right side >	Hold on right side >	Hold on each side >	Hold >	Hold >
BEGINNER 30 secs	BEGINNER 30 secs	BEGINNER 30 secs/side	BEGINNER 30 secs	BEGINNER 45 secs
ADVANCED 45 secs	ADVANCED 45 secs	ADVANCED 60 secs/side	ADVANCED 60 secs	ADVANCED 75 secs

GOOD FOR

• Athletes and fitness enthusiasts who want to improve overall performance

• Those who want to build and tone the muscles in the hips, glutes, and thighs

• People who want to prevent knee and back injury

• Anyone who wants a challenging yoga workout

GUIDELINES

• Hold the postures for the time given, breathing consciously to work deeper into the poses.

• If the instructions say to hold on each side, do the left side and then the right side in succession.

• Move as fluidly as possible from one posture to the next without resetting to a starting position unless necessary.

• Push yourself, go deeper, and hold each posture for the time given. When your legs start shaking, just breathe and keep holding it until the end.

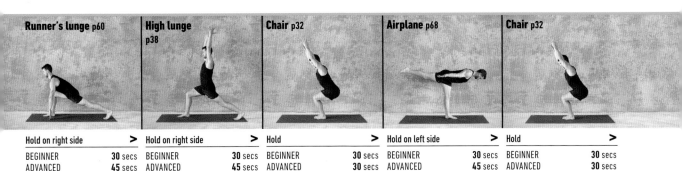

Runner's lunge p60		**High lunge** p38		**Chair** p32		**Airplane** p68		**Chair** p32	
Hold on right side	>	Hold on right side	>	Hold	>	Hold on left side	>	Hold	>
BEGINNER	**30** secs	BEGINNER	**30** secs	BEGINNER	**30** secs	BEGINNER	**30** secs	BEGINNER	**30** secs
ADVANCED	**45** secs	ADVANCED	**45** secs	ADVANCED	**30** secs	ADVANCED	**45** secs	ADVANCED	**30** secs

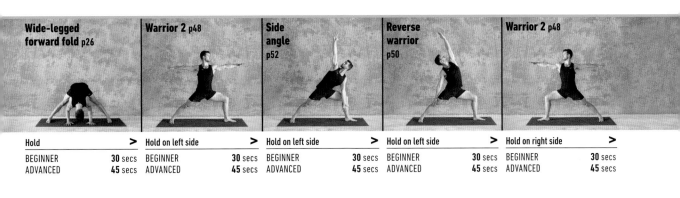

Wide-legged forward fold p26		**Warrior 2** p48		**Side angle** p52		**Reverse warrior** p50		**Warrior 2** p48	
Hold	>	Hold on left side	>	Hold on left side	>	Hold on left side	>	Hold on right side	>
BEGINNER	**30** secs	BEGINNER	**30** secs	BEGINNER	**30** secs	BEGINNER	**30** secs	BEGINNER	**30** secs
ADVANCED	**45** secs	ADVANCED	**45** secs	ADVANCED	**45** secs	ADVANCED	**45** secs	ADVANCED	**45** secs

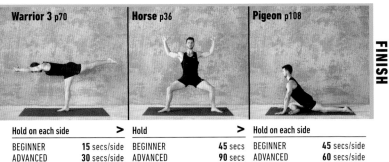

FINISH

Warrior 3 p70		**Horse** p36		**Pigeon** p108	
Hold on each side	>	Hold	>	Hold on each side	
BEGINNER	**15** secs/side	BEGINNER	**45** secs	BEGINNER	**45** secs/side
ADVANCED	**30** secs/side	ADVANCED	**90** secs	ADVANCED	**60** secs/side

ACTIVE HIP MOBILITY
FOR STRENGTH, POWER, AND CONTROL

Ever wonder how martial artists can kick so high, and continue to hold their leg up? It starts with active hip mobility. This workout challenges you to build strength in your extreme range of motion, to achieve a new level of power in your hips, elevate your athletic performance, and take your endurance to new heights.

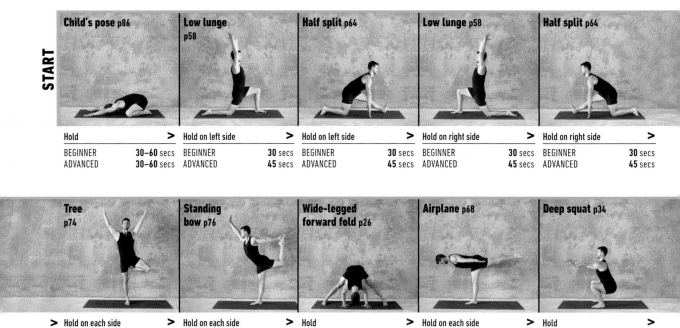

START

Child's pose p86

Hold >

| BEGINNER | 30–60 secs |
| ADVANCED | 30–60 secs |

Low lunge p58

Hold on left side >

| BEGINNER | 30 secs |
| ADVANCED | 45 secs |

Half split p64

Hold on left side >

| BEGINNER | 30 secs |
| ADVANCED | 45 secs |

Low lunge p58

Hold on right side >

| BEGINNER | 30 secs |
| ADVANCED | 45 secs |

Half split p64

Hold on right side >

| BEGINNER | 30 secs |
| ADVANCED | 45 secs |

Tree p74

> Hold on each side >

| BEGINNER | 30 secs/side |
| ADVANCED | 45 secs/side |

Standing bow p76

Hold on each side >

| BEGINNER | 30 secs/side |
| ADVANCED | 45 secs/side |

Wide-legged forward fold p26

Hold >

| BEGINNER | 30 secs |
| ADVANCED | 45 secs |

Airplane p68

Hold on each side >

| BEGINNER | 30 secs/side |
| ADVANCED | 45 secs/side |

Deep squat p34

Hold >

| BEGINNER | 30 secs |
| ADVANCED | 45 secs |

Frog p110

> Hold >

| BEGINNER | 90 secs |
| ADVANCED | 120 secs |

Hamstring strap stretch p118

Hold on each side >

| BEGINNER | 45 secs/side |
| ADVANCED | 60 secs/side |

Inner-thigh strap stretch p120

Hold on each side >

| BEGINNER | 45 secs/side |
| ADVANCED | 45 secs/side |

Outer-thigh strap stretch p122

Hold on each side

| BEGINNER | 45 secs/side |
| ADVANCED | 45 secs/side |

FINISH

GOOD FOR

• Athletes, martial artists, and fitness enthusiasts who want to significantly improve hip mobility

• Anyone who wants a challenging yoga workout

• Strengthening the lower body for advanced movements or gymnastics

YOU WILL NEED

• a strap

GUIDELINES

• Hold the postures for the time given, breathing consciously to work deeper into the poses.

• If the instructions say to hold on each side, do the left side and then the right side in succession.

• Move as fluidly as possible from one posture to the next without resetting to a starting position unless necessary.

• You'll get the most from this routine by trying to reach your maximum depth in each posture, working on strength and mobility at the same time.

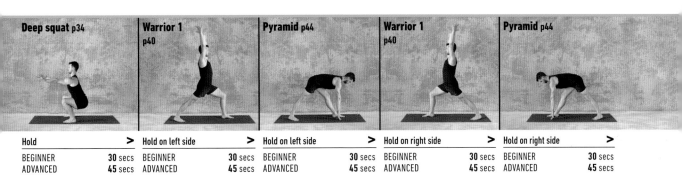

Deep squat p34

Hold >

| BEGINNER | 30 secs |
| ADVANCED | 45 secs |

Warrior 1 p40

Hold on left side >

| BEGINNER | 30 secs |
| ADVANCED | 45 secs |

Pyramid p44

Hold on left side >

| BEGINNER | 30 secs |
| ADVANCED | 45 secs |

Warrior 1 p40

Hold on right side >

| BEGINNER | 30 secs |
| ADVANCED | 45 secs |

Pyramid p44

Hold on right side >

| BEGINNER | 30 secs |
| ADVANCED | 45 secs |

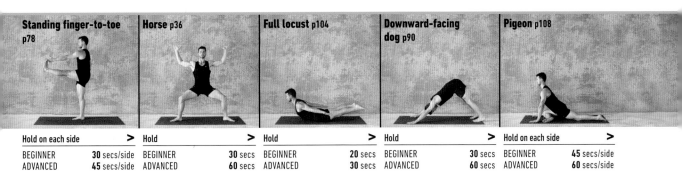

Standing finger-to-toe p78

Hold on each side >

| BEGINNER | 30 secs/side |
| ADVANCED | 45 secs/side |

Horse p36

Hold >

| BEGINNER | 30 secs |
| ADVANCED | 60 secs |

Full locust p104

Hold >

| BEGINNER | 20 secs |
| ADVANCED | 30 secs |

Downward-facing dog p90

Hold >

| BEGINNER | 30 secs |
| ADVANCED | 60 secs |

Pigeon p108

Hold on each side >

| BEGINNER | 45 secs/side |
| ADVANCED | 60 secs/side |

ANKLE MOBILITY
AND INJURY PREVENTION

It's an often overlooked aspect of fitness, but you'll be surprised by what a modest increase in ankle mobility can do for your movement. It helps prevent injury in the ankles, knees, hips, and spine. This is a fantastic routine to improve squats, strengthen the body as a runner, and boost performance in any sport.

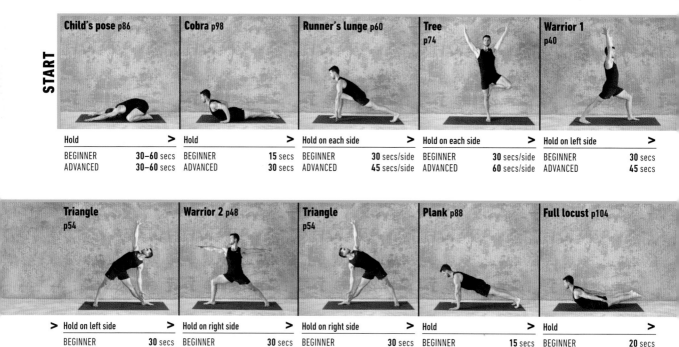

START

Child's pose p86	Cobra p98	Runner's lunge p60	Tree p74	Warrior 1 p40
Hold >	Hold >	Hold on each side >	Hold on each side >	Hold on left side >
BEGINNER 30–60 secs	BEGINNER 15 secs	BEGINNER 30 secs/side	BEGINNER 30 secs/side	BEGINNER 30 secs
ADVANCED 30–60 secs	ADVANCED 30 secs	ADVANCED 45 secs/side	ADVANCED 60 secs/side	ADVANCED 45 secs

Triangle p54	Warrior 2 p48	Triangle p54	Plank p88	Full locust p104
> Hold on left side >	Hold on right side >	Hold on right side >	Hold >	Hold >
BEGINNER 30 secs	BEGINNER 30 secs	BEGINNER 30 secs	BEGINNER 15 secs	BEGINNER 20 secs
ADVANCED 45 secs	ADVANCED 45 secs	ADVANCED 45 secs	ADVANCED 15 secs	ADVANCED 30 secs

GOOD FOR

- Athletes and fitness enthusiasts to prevent knee and ankle injury
- Runners, triathletes, and swimmers
- People with a history of ankle problems
- Weight lifters and functional fitness enthusiasts

GUIDELINES

- Hold the postures for the time given, breathing consciously to work deeper into the poses.
- If the instructions say to hold on each side, do the left side and then the right side in succession.
- Move as fluidly as possible from one posture to the next without resetting to a starting position unless necessary.
- Your ankles don't open up as quickly as your shoulders or hips, so you'll have to work a little harder to see results.

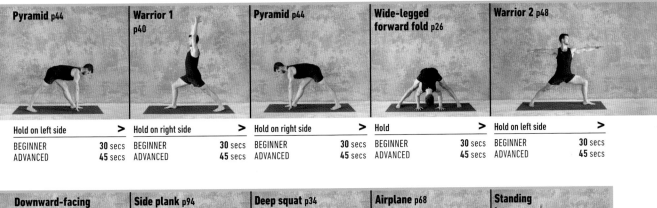

Pyramid p44

Hold on left side >

BEGINNER	**30** secs
ADVANCED	**45** secs

Warrior 1 p40

Hold on right side >

BEGINNER	**30** secs
ADVANCED	**45** secs

Pyramid p44

Hold on right side >

BEGINNER	**30** secs
ADVANCED	**45** secs

Wide-legged forward fold p26

Hold >

BEGINNER	**30** secs
ADVANCED	**45** secs

Warrior 2 p48

Hold on left side >

BEGINNER	**30** secs
ADVANCED	**45** secs

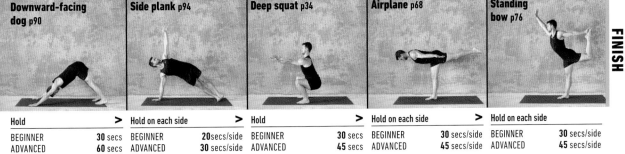

Downward-facing dog p90

Hold >

BEGINNER	**30** secs
ADVANCED	**60** secs

Side plank p94

Hold on each side >

BEGINNER	**20**secs/side
ADVANCED	**30** secs/side

Deep squat p34

Hold >

BEGINNER	**30** secs
ADVANCED	**45** secs

Airplane p68

Hold on each side >

BEGINNER	**30** secs/side
ADVANCED	**45** secs/side

Standing bow p76

Hold on each side

BEGINNER	**30** secs/side
ADVANCED	**45** secs/side

FINISH

BALANCE FOR BEGINNERS

Before improving balance, you first need to ensure you're using all the correct muscles. This beginner's workout starts with postures to warm-up your core and activate the muscles used to balance, then advances to the best balance postures. It takes practice and patience, but doing this routine regularly will improve this skill with time.

START

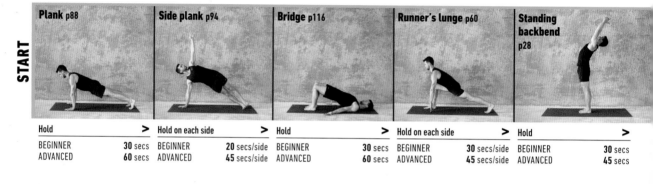

Plank p88	Side plank p94	Bridge p116	Runner's lunge p60	Standing backbend p28
Hold >	**Hold on each side** >	**Hold** >	**Hold on each side** >	**Hold** >
BEGINNER 30 secs	BEGINNER 20 secs/side	BEGINNER 30 secs	BEGINNER 30 secs/side	BEGINNER 30 secs
ADVANCED 60 secs	ADVANCED 45 secs/side	ADVANCED 60 secs	ADVANCED 45 secs/side	ADVANCED 45 secs

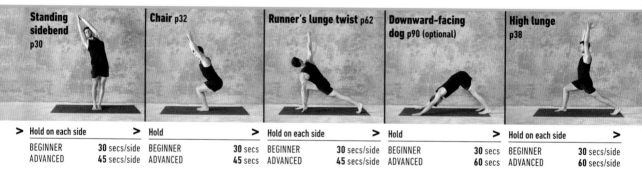

Standing sidebend p30	Chair p32	Runner's lunge twist p62	Downward-facing dog p90 (optional)	High lunge p38
> **Hold on each side** >	**Hold** >	**Hold on each side** >	**Hold** >	**Hold on each side** >
BEGINNER 30 secs/side	BEGINNER 30 secs	BEGINNER 30 secs/side	BEGINNER 30 secs	BEGINNER 30 secs/side
ADVANCED 45 secs/side	ADVANCED 45 secs	ADVANCED 45 secs/side	ADVANCED 60 secs	ADVANCED 60 secs/side

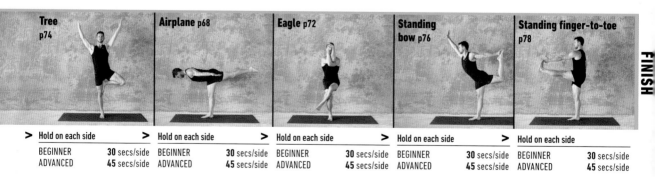

Tree p74	Airplane p68	Eagle p72	Standing bow p76	Standing finger-to-toe p78
> **Hold on each side** >	**Hold on each side** >	**Hold on each side** >	**Hold on each side** >	**Hold on each side**
BEGINNER 30 secs/side	BEGINNER 30 secs/side	BEGINNER 30 secs/side	BEGINNER 30 secs/side	BEGINNER 30 secs/side
ADVANCED 45 secs/side	ADVANCED 45 secs/side	ADVANCED 45 secs/side	ADVANCED 45 secs/side	ADVANCED 45 secs/side

FINISH

GOOD FOR

• Anyone who needs greater balance and body awareness

• People of all fitness levels to strengthen the hips, legs, core, and ankles

• Anyone interested in injury prevention, regardless of physical activity

• Those who want to develop lower-body strength and endurance with minimal strain on the joints

GUIDELINES

• Hold the postures for the time given, breathing consciously to work deeper into the poses.

• If the instructions say to hold on each side, do the left side and then the right side in succession.

• Balance is all about controlling your breathing and intently focusing on what you're doing with your body. Stare at a non-moving point to help you achieve balance in the postures. If you lose your balance, slowly get back into it with control.

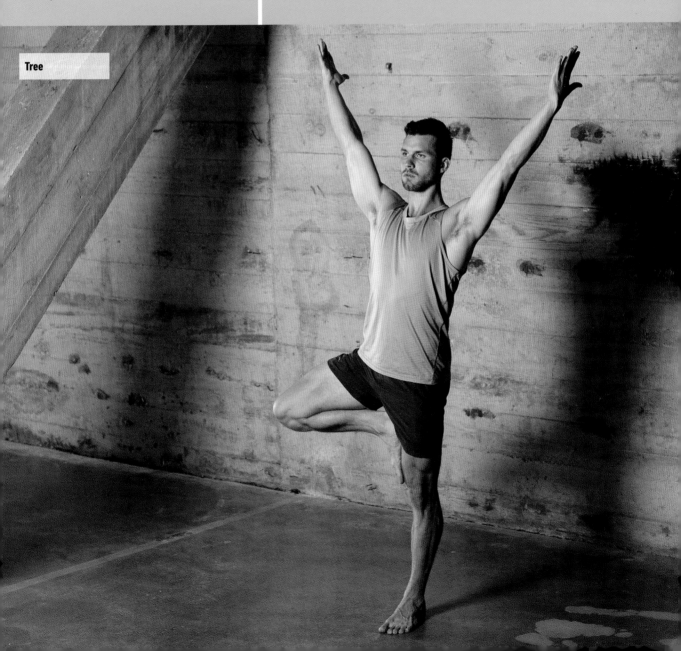

Tree

NEXT-LEVEL BALANCE

This advanced workout challenges you to improve balance, strength, and mobility with the most difficult balance postures this book offers—it's for those who already have strong body awareness. Standing on one leg while testing mobility is immensely demanding, and improves muscle activation, strength, and flexibility, while helping prevent injury.

START

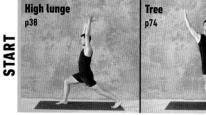

High lunge p38
Tree p74
Airplane p68
Standing bow p76
Eagle p72

Hold on each side >
BEGINNER	**45** secs/side
ADVANCED	**60** secs/side

Hold on each side, then repeat >
BEGINNER	**30** secs/side
ADVANCED	**60** secs/side

Hold on each side, then repeat >
BEGINNER	**30** secs/side
ADVANCED	**60** secs/side

Hold on each side, then repeat >
BEGINNER	**30** secs/side
ADVANCED	**60** secs/side

Hold on each side, then repeat >
BEGINNER	**30** secs/side
ADVANCED	**60** secs/side

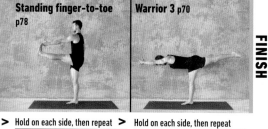

Standing finger-to-toe p78
Warrior 3 p70

FINISH

> Hold on each side, then repeat >
BEGINNER	**30** secs/side
ADVANCED	**60** secs/side

Hold on each side, then repeat
BEGINNER	**30** secs/side
ADVANCED	**60** secs/side

GOOD FOR

• Athletes, runners, and fitness enthusiasts who want to improve overall performance

• Anybody who wants a challenging yoga routine

• People who need a very efficient workout in a short amount of time

• Those with an advanced fitness level

GUIDELINES

• Hold the postures for the time given, breathing consciously to work deeper into the poses.

• This routine is structured differently than the others. Do High lunge once on each side to warm up. Then do each posture twice on both sides before proceeding to the next.

• Start off slow, easing into each pose to gradually work deeper into it. Since you're doing each one twice, you have time to build up to your best expression of each posture.

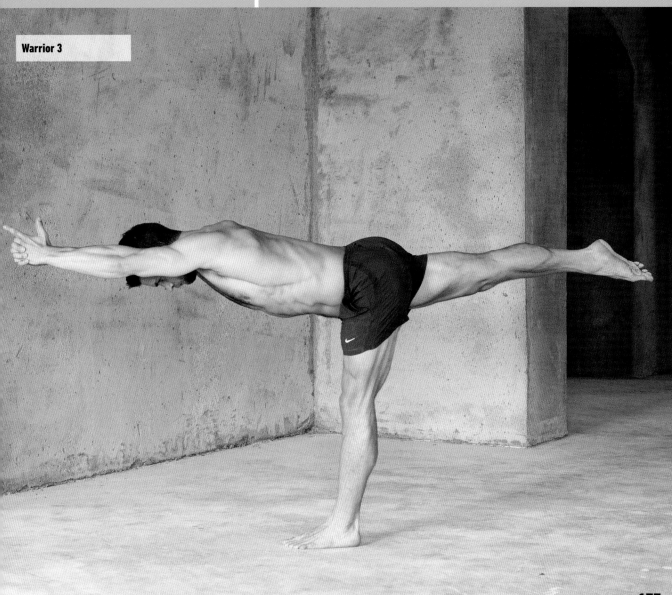

Warrior 3

POWERFUL TWISTS

Movements involving quick changes in direction, throwing, dodging, and swinging all require mobility and power in a twist. The more range of motion you have in your spine and hips, the more force you generate in rotational movements. Performance aside, spinal strength and mobility are important for longevity and preventing injury.

START

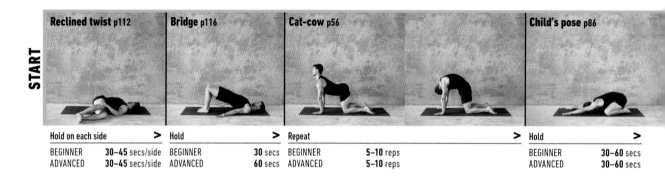

Reclined twist p112		Bridge p116		Cat-cow p56				Child's pose p86	
Hold on each side >		**Hold** >		**Repeat**			>	**Hold** >	
BEGINNER	30–45 secs/side	BEGINNER	30 secs	BEGINNER	5–10 reps			BEGINNER	30–60 secs
ADVANCED	30–45 secs/side	ADVANCED	60 secs	ADVANCED	5–10 reps			ADVANCED	30–60 secs

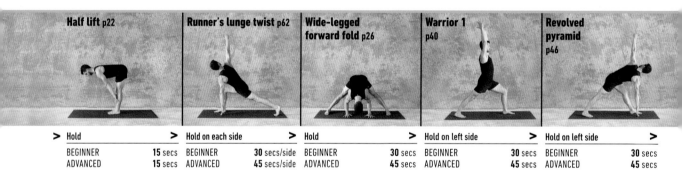

Half lift p22		Runner's lunge twist p62		Wide-legged forward fold p26		Warrior 1 p40		Revolved pyramid p46	
> **Hold** >		**Hold on each side** >		**Hold** >		**Hold on left side** >		**Hold on left side** >	
BEGINNER	15 secs	BEGINNER	30 secs/side	BEGINNER	30 secs	BEGINNER	30 secs	BEGINNER	30 secs
ADVANCED	15 secs	ADVANCED	45 secs/side	ADVANCED	45 secs	ADVANCED	45 secs	ADVANCED	45 secs

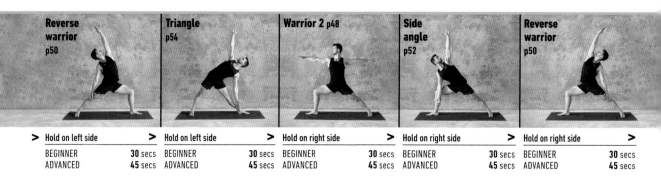

Reverse warrior p50		Triangle p54		Warrior 2 p48		Side angle p52		Reverse warrior p50	
> **Hold on left side** >		**Hold on left side** >		**Hold on right side** >		**Hold on right side** >		**Hold on right side** >	
BEGINNER	30 secs	BEGINNER	30 secs	BEGINNER	30 secs	BEGINNER	30 secs	BEGINNER	30 secs
ADVANCED	45 secs	ADVANCED	45 secs	ADVANCED	45 secs	ADVANCED	45 secs	ADVANCED	45 secs

GOOD FOR

• Anyone who infrequently moves their spine throughout the day

• Rotational athletes (for sports such as baseball, hockey, golf, tennis, lacrosse, and swimming)

• People with postural issues, spine curvature issues, or chronic back pain

• Anyone prone to back injury (but is healthy at the time of doing this routine)

GUIDELINES

• Hold the postures for the time given, or repeat for the reps given, breathing consciously to work deeper into the poses.

• If the instructions say to hold on each side, do the left side and then the right side in succession.

• Move as fluidly as possible from one posture to the next without resetting to a starting position unless necessary.

• For safety, use your breath to optimize the movement. Always inhale first to lengthen your spine as much as possible, then exhale to deepen the twist, bend, or fold.

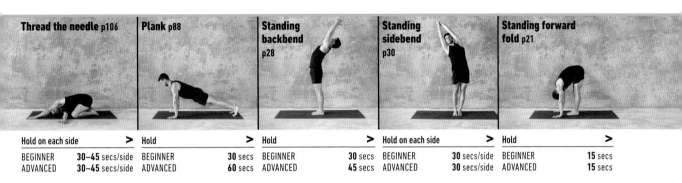

Thread the needle p106		Plank p88		Standing backbend p28		Standing sidebend p30		Standing forward fold p21	
Hold on each side	>	**Hold**	>	**Hold**	>	**Hold on each side**	>	**Hold**	>
BEGINNER	**30–45** secs/side	BEGINNER	**30** secs	BEGINNER	**30** secs	BEGINNER	**30** secs/side	BEGINNER	**15** secs
ADVANCED	**30–45** secs/side	ADVANCED	**60** secs	ADVANCED	**45** secs	ADVANCED	**30** secs/side	ADVANCED	**15** secs

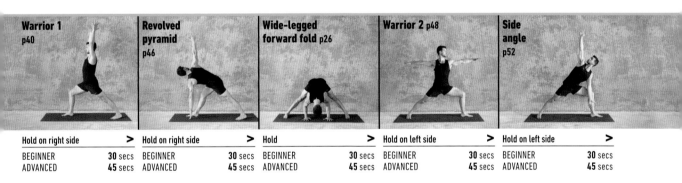

Warrior 1 p40		Revolved pyramid p46		Wide-legged forward fold p26		Warrior 2 p48		Side angle p52	
Hold on right side	>	**Hold on right side**	>	**Hold**	>	**Hold on left side**	>	**Hold on left side**	>
BEGINNER	**30** secs	BEGINNER	**30** secs	BEGINNER	**30** secs	BEGINNER	**30** secs	BEGINNER	**30** secs
ADVANCED	**45** secs	ADVANCED	**45** secs	ADVANCED	**45** secs	ADVANCED	**45** secs	ADVANCED	**45** secs

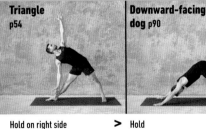

Triangle p54		Downward-facing dog p90	
Hold on right side	>	**Hold**	
BEGINNER	**30** secs	BEGINNER	**30** secs
ADVANCED	**45** secs	ADVANCED	**60** secs

FINISH

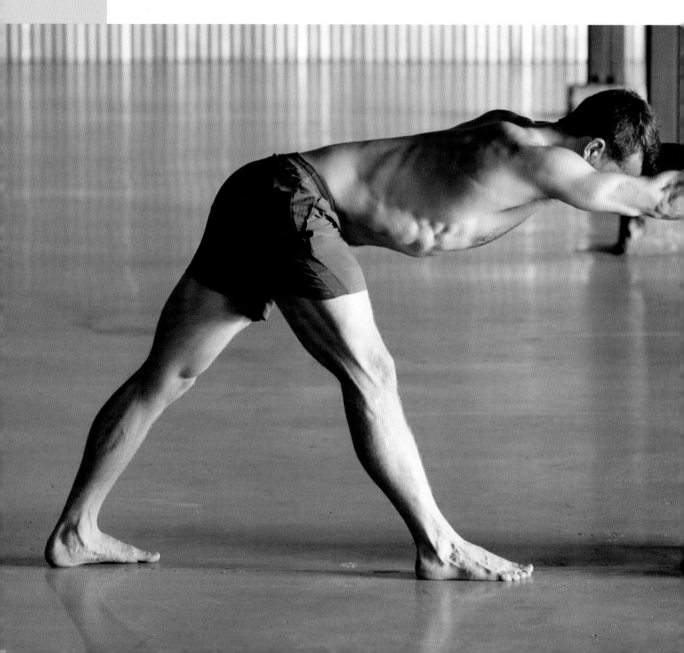

3 PROGRAMS

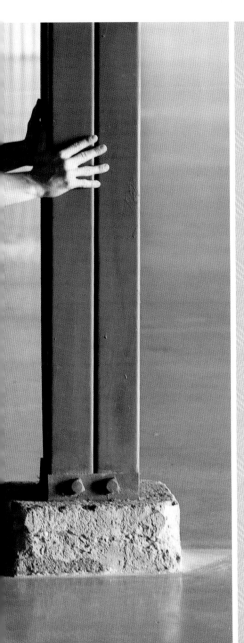

Follow a plan, and you will notice improvement. Choose one of these three distinct, multi-week programs, and be confident you can expect results.

12 weeks for general fitness

This program helps you improve strength, mobility, and balance; relieve chronic aches and pains; improve posture and energy levels; build and tone muscles; and burn fat.

12 weeks for athletic performance

Pair this performance-focused program with your existing workout program to increase mobility, improve muscle activation, move more fluidly, decrease recovery time, and reduce your risk of injury.

16 weeks for a healthy spine and core

This functional yoga program helps you recover or prevent injury in your spine, and drastically reduces lower-back, neck, and other spine-related pain. Strengthen your core, increase hip strength and mobility, and improve posture, too.

12 WEEKS FOR
GENERAL FITNESS

This program helps you establish a habit of daily yoga workouts while improving your overall fitness. You'll fix your posture, improve your overall physical well-being, and develop a solid foundation of strength and mobility. Workouts build in difficulty as the program progresses, so you stay challenged as your body gets stronger.

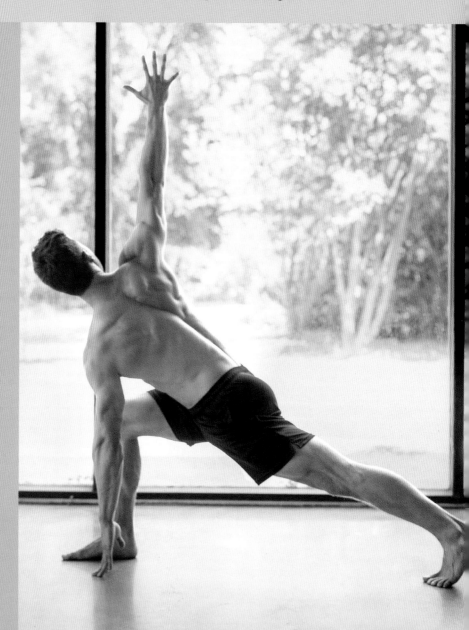

GOOD FOR

- Improving general fitness
- Developing functional movement for day-to-day tasks
- Improving energy levels, getting better sleep, and boosting overall health and mental well-being

GUIDELINES

- For each phase, complete the 1-week sequence 4 times for a total of 4 weeks.
- If you miss a workout, don't skip it completely—just pick up the next day where you left off, or double up on workouts the following day.
- It's okay if a phase takes you longer than 4 weeks, but don't move on until you complete it.
- Only move on to the next phase if you can complete 90 percent of each workout.

PHASE 1: WEEKS 1–4

DAY 1 — Foundational core strength
p156

DAY 2 — Hip strength and mobility essentials
p166

DAY 3 — Basic shoulder strength and mobility
p162

DAY 4 — Essential hip mobility
p148

DAY 5 — Strong spine, strong body
p160

DAY 6 — Balance for beginners
p174

DAY 7 — Rest day

PHASE 2: WEEKS 5–8

DAY 1 — Foundational core strength
p156

DAY 2 — Ankle mobility and injury prevention
p172

DAY 3 — Balance for beginners
p174

DAY 4 — Powerful twists
p178

DAY 5 — Posture fixer-upper
p144

DAY 6 — Basic shoulder strength and mobility
p162

DAY 7 — Rest day

PHASE 3: WEEKS 9–12

DAY 1 — Abs on fire
p158

DAY 2 — Strong hips challenge
p168

DAY 3 — Next-level balance
p176

DAY 4 — Too much sitting
p152

DAY 5 — Active hip mobility for strength, power, and control
p170

DAY 6 — Total-body strength
p150

DAY 7 — Rest day

12 WEEKS FOR
ATHLETIC PERFORMANCE

This program is ideal for endurance athletes, serious runners, or other competitive athletes to combine with their existing regimen. The days alternate between strength and mobility workouts. Try to schedule the mobility workouts (odd-numbered days) on the same days as your non-yoga workouts.

GOOD FOR

• Improving mobility, balance, and body control

• Decreasing recovery time and reducing soreness

• More effective breathing and cardiovascular strength

• Strengthening core, spine, hips, and areas neglected by other workouts

• Preventing soft-tissue injuries

GUIDELINES

• For each phase, complete the 1-week sequence 4 times for a total of 4 weeks.

• If you miss a workout, don't skip it completely—just pick up the next day where you left off, or double up on workouts the following day.

• Cool down each day with one of the restorative workouts (see pp130–141).

• It's okay if a phase takes you longer than 4 weeks, but don't move on until you complete it.

• Only move on to the next phase if you can complete 90 percent of each workout.

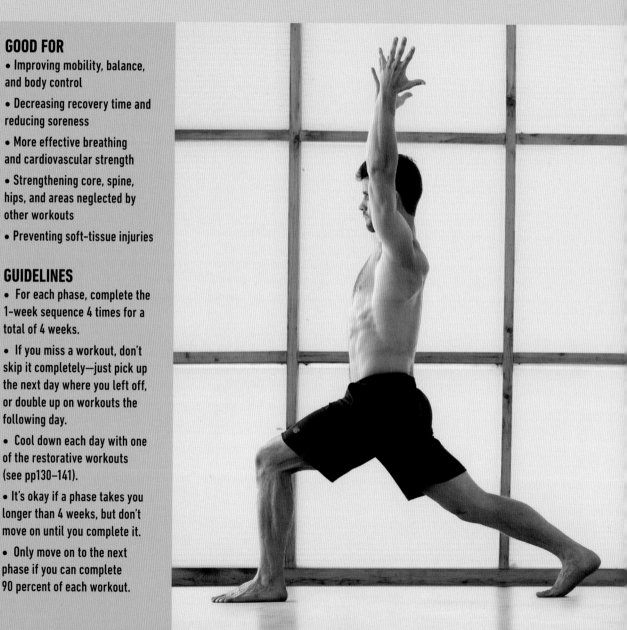

PHASE 1: WEEKS 1–4

DAY 1
Hip strength and mobility essentials
p166

DAY 2
Essential hip mobility
p148

DAY 3
Foundational core strength
p156

DAY 4
Ankle mobility and injury prevention
p172

DAY 5
Strong spine, strong body
p160

DAY 6
Balance for beginners
p174

DAY 7
Basic shoulder strength and mobility
p162

PHASE 2: WEEKS 5–8

DAY 1
Balance for beginners
p174

DAY 2
Active hip mobility for strength, power, and control
p170

DAY 3
Posture fixer-upper
p144

DAY 4
Powerful twists
p178

DAY 5
Standing relief
p142

DAY 6
Basic shoulder strength and mobility
p162

DAY 7
Total-body strength
p150

PHASE 3: WEEKS 9–12

DAY 1
Too much sitting
p152

DAY 2
Strong hips challenge
p168

DAY 3
Total-body strength
p150

DAY 4
Advanced upper-body work for bulletproof shoulders
p164

DAY 5
Foundational core strength
p156

DAY 6
Powerful twists
p178

DAY 7
Next-level balance
p176

16 WEEKS FOR A
HEALTHY SPINE AND CORE

Use this program to aid recovery from back injury or surgery, restore balance to your spine, and experience everyday life without chronic back pain. These workouts help you establish a daily habit of yoga, while strengthening the weaknesses and correcting the movement patterns that are the root of back pain.

GOOD FOR

- Building foundational strength and mobility, especially in the spine

- Preventing or recovering from a back injury

- Relieving daily aches and pain

GUIDELINES

- For each phase, complete the 2-week sequence 4 times for a total of 8 weeks.

- If you miss a workout, don't skip it completely—just pick up the next day where you left off, or double up on workouts the following day.

- It's okay if a phase takes you longer than 8 weeks, but don't move on until you complete it.

- Only move on to the next phase if you can complete 90 percent of each workout.

NOTE: This program complements physical therapy, but it does not replace it. If you feel sharp pain, numbness, or tingling, seek medical advice.

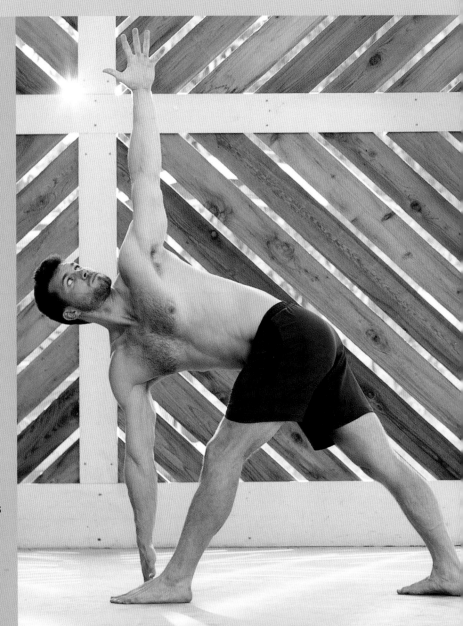

PHASE 1: WEEKS 1–8

DAY 1	**Strong spine, strong body** p160	**DAY 8**	**Standing relief** p142
DAY 2	**Hip strength and mobility essentials** p166	**DAY 9**	**Back pain relief** p134
DAY 3	**Essential hip mobility** p148	**DAY 10**	**Posture fixer-upper** p144
DAY 4	**Balance for beginners** p174	**DAY 11**	**Balance for beginners** p174
DAY 5	**Total-body soreness relief** p132	**DAY 12**	**Standing relief** p142
DAY 6	**Foundational core strength** p156	**DAY 13**	**Strong spine, strong body** p160
DAY 7	**Stiff neck relief** p146	**DAY 14**	**Stiff neck relief** p146

PHASE 2: WEEKS 9–16

DAY 1	**Foundational core strength** p156	**DAY 8**	**Total-body soreness relief** p132
DAY 2	**Strong spine, strong body** p160	**DAY 9**	**Powerful twists** p178
DAY 3	**Balance for beginners** p174	**DAY 10**	**Standing relief** p142
DAY 4	**Stiff neck relief** p146	**DAY 11**	**Balance for beginners** p174
DAY 5	**Posture fixer-upper** p144	**DAY 12**	**Posture fixer-upper** p144
DAY 6	**Active hip mobility for strength, power, and control** p170	**DAY 13**	**Stiff neck relief** p146
DAY 7	**Too much sitting** p152	**DAY 14**	**Too much sitting** p152

INDEX

ABOUT THE AUTHOR

Dean Pohlman is the leader of the number-one brand of men's yoga for fitness, Man Flow Yoga. Since starting it in 2013, he has published an e-book, *Yoga Basics for Men*, released a DVD, *Yoga Boost*, and built an audience of over 150,000 on social media. Dean's work has been used by professional athletes in the National Football League and Major League Lacrosse.

Dean's fitness-centric approach to yoga allows thousands of men who would not otherwise try yoga to get stronger, improve mobility, and prevent injury. His unique, strength-focused approach helps people experience atypical results when compared to traditional yoga, including increased muscle mass, improved muscle activation, and increased active range of motion.

AUTHOR'S THANKS

First off, I would like to thank Alpha and DK for the opportunity to write this book. Thank you to Alexandra Elliott, editor, and Nigel Wright, art director for photography, for coming to Austin to conduct the photo shoot (and eat Texas BBQ and breakfast tacos), as well as to Ann Barton, co-editor, for the wonderful feedback throughout the entire writing process.

I'd also like to acknowledge my parents, Brad and Julie, for allowing me to pursue my mission of improving people's fitness through yoga without judgment. Finally, I'd like to thank everyone who helped to grow Man Flow Yoga from a YouTube channel into a movement. Whether you're someone I trained via webcam, a member of the Man Flow Yoga Members' Area, or if you just happened to like a post on social media, thank you!

PUBLISHER'S THANKS

Proofreader: Laura Caddell
Indexer: Brad Herriman
Digital technician for photography: Robert G. Gomez

Editor: Alexandra Elliott
Senior editors: Ann Barton and Kathryn Meeker
Book designer: Hannah Moore
Senior art editor: Glenda Fisher
Art director for photography: Nigel Wright
Photographer: Dennis Burnett
Jacket designer: Steve Marsden
Managing editor: Stephanie Farrow
Managing art editor: Christine Keilty
Publisher: Mike Sanders

First American Edition, 2018
Published in the United States by DK Publishing
6081 E. 82nd Street, Indianapolis, Indiana 46250

Copyright © 2018 Dorling Kindersley Limited
A Penguin Random House Company
19 20 21 22   10 9 8 7 6 5 4
009–309802–May/2018

ISBN: 978-1-4654-7348-6

Library of Congress Catalog Number: 2017956773

Note: This publication contains the opinions and ideas of its author(s). It is intended to provide helpful and informative material on
the subject matter covered. It is sold with the understanding that the author(s) and publisher are not engaged in rendering
professional services in the book. If the reader requires personal assistance or advice, a competent professional should be
consulted. The author(s) and publisher specifically disclaim any responsibility for any liability, loss, or risk, personal or otherwise,
which is incurred as a consequence, directly or indirectly, of the use and application of any of the contents of this book.

Trademarks: All terms mentioned in this book that are known to be or are suspected of being trademarks or service marks have
been appropriately capitalized. Alpha Books, DK, and Penguin Random House LLC cannot attest to the accuracy of this
information. Use of a term in this book should not be regarded as affecting the validity of any trademark or service mark.

DK books are available at special discounts when purchased in bulk for sales promotions, premiums, fund-raising, or educational
use. For details, contact: DK Publishing Special Markets, 1450 Broadway, Suite 801, New York, NY 10018 or SpecialSales@dk.com.

Printed and bound in China

All images © Dorling Kindersley Limited
For further information see: www.dkimages.com

A WORLD OF IDEAS:
SEE ALL THERE IS TO KNOW

www.dk.com